Music Therapy

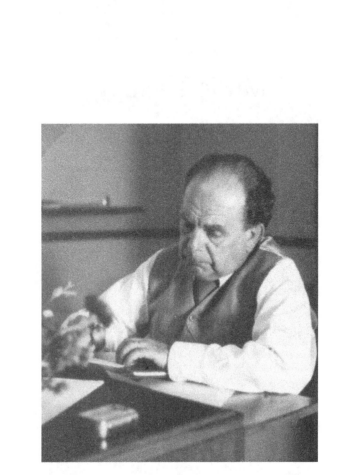

Karl König in Camphill, 1960

Music Therapy

Research and Insights

Karl König

Edited by Katarina Seeherr

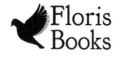
Floris Books

Content warning

This book was mostly written between the 1940s and 1960s and includes extracts of historical texts from the 19th century onwards. It reflects an understanding of disabilities from past eras and contains language that, although widely used to describe disabled people in those times, is no longer acceptable and may be shocking for modern readers. Some extracts also include gendered terms that would not be used today. We recommend reading this book with an understanding of the contexts in which it was written.

Karl König Archive, Vol. 23
Subject: Medicine

Series editor: Richard Steel

Karl König's collected works are issued by
the Karl König Institute, Aberdeen

First published in English by Floris Books in 2024
© 2024 Trustees of the Karl König Institute

e Also available as an eBook

British Library CIP Data available
ISBN 978-178250-892-2

Contents

Letters

Notebooks

Introduction: Karl König as Musician, Researcher and Therapist

Katarina Seeherr

It is not easy to express music in words, yet this volume is an attempt to publish documents which, in part, have been stored in the Karl König Archive for a long time, but will hopefully resonate with those who are open to the healing effects of music. This introduction describes the birth process of anthroposophical music therapy within the framework of König's musical biography. At the beginning of this development there is König himself as he experienced music or was actively making music. Over time, however, he came to understand the healing effect that music can have, and that music is concretely related to the human being. Many musicians, both during König's lifetime and since, have sensed his enthusiasm and felt inspired to create new, healing compositions with sounds, tones and movements. They have developed new skills, formed research circles and devised training courses that carry the original impulse into the world in ever new guises. They have become music therapists.

Karl König was born on September 25, 1902, in Vienna as the only child of Adolf Ber König and Bertha König. He appears to have been an intellectually precocious child. He read a lot, collecting a large library early on, which included works by Schiller, Goethe, Schopenhauer and Kant. He was also very musical. He received piano lessons, which he loved, and had an Ehrbach grand piano in his room because his mother was of the opinion that he was already playing quite well.[1]

In a diary entry from 1918, König described how he had discovered music the year before at the age of fifteen:

> There was a major turning point in my relationship to music in Autumn 1917. I do not know how it happened, but I had not been to the opera for two years. Then I bought a ticket to [Wagner's] *The Mastersinger,* and what I felt there is indescribable. It was the first major work of music I had heard. When it was over I went for a long walk – for two hours – because there was such turmoil inside me. I would say that I was full to overflowing. From that moment on, music became of the highest importance to me.

After this, König went to the opera every week, enjoying the musical life of Vienna to the full:

> I saw almost all of Wagner's operas and musical dramas: *The Mastersinger* with Slezak, the *Götterdämmerung* with Weidt as Brunhilde, *Rheingold, The Flying Dutchman, Tannhäuser* and *Lohengrin.*[2]

He then lists more operas he had seen, still at the age of fifteen: *Don Giovanni, The Magic Flute, Don Juan, The Merry Widows of Windsor, Fidelio, Aida, Carmen, Martha,* and *Troubadour.* Only a couple of months had passed between his discovery of his love for music as described in the diary entry above and this list. When he was sixteen, he wrote that he had seen Richard Wagner's Ring Cycle twice but *Siegfried* only once. He went to symphonic concerts, and a classmate played all of Beethoven's symphonies for him on the piano, as well as Wagner's *Siegfried* and *Tristan and Isolde*. König thus had an extraordinarily rich experience of music already by the age of sixteen. A classmate put some poems König had written to music and these newly composed songs were played to him by one classmate playing the piano, another the violin, and a third singing.[3]

Of the many composers he loved, König related especially to Ludwig van Beethoven, Richard Wagner, Gustav Mahler and Johann Sebastian Bach. Mahler, whose time as concertmaster in Vienna (1897–1907) König had missed because he was too young, remained a special inspiration to him throughout his life.

On May 18, 1921, the tenth anniversary of Mahler's death, König visited Mahler's grave with his best friend, Alfred Bergel. When he visited Mahler's grave again in October 1963 and looked back on this moment, König realised that it had taken place at the time of his first moon node when he was eighteen years old.[4] This is why he had added to the diary entry for that day: 'The tenth anniversary of Mahler's death. Conclusion of the first moon node.'

The experience König had soon after his first moon node made a deep and lasting impression on him. König's biographical essay celebrating Mahler's one-hundredth birthday, written in 1960, describes Mahler's life in a very sensitive way.[5] A photograph of the great composer and conductor hung in his room in Scotland. König got to know Mahler's wife, Alma Mahler-Werfel, in Paris during his escape from the Nazi regime. He also corresponded with Mahler's student and admirer Bruno Walter, who conducted concerts in Vienna during König's time there, and who later found his way to anthroposophy. König's mother, Bertha König, came from Iglau in Mähren, where Mahler had spent his childhood and adolescence.

For a long time König debated whether to become a musical conductor before finally choosing the medical profession and then, later on, curative education.

Christof-Andreas Lindenberg relates an anecdote in which Ferdinand Rauter, one of the first Camphill musicians and later a famous pianist in London, said of König with a wink:

> When König was still not sure whether he wanted to study medicine or become a conductor, he had a vision at Mahler's graveside where he thought he heard Mahler say: 'In God's name, do not become a musician, stay in medicine!'[6]

Thus König found his mission as a physician.

The mystery of life and music

Throughout his life, König was occupied with the theme of life forces. During his medical studies he gave a lecture called 'The Science of Living Things' at the Institute for Embryology in Vienna on December 3, 1925. In it he said that the natural sciences had emerged just as the more intuitive forms of knowledge about nature were receding. He said that philosophy was the precursor to natural science and that, according to Socrates, before philosophy came amazement. Being amazed is the longing for lost knowledge:

> In Goethe there still lived this amazement about the living force, which helped him to roughly fathom the basic principles of the structure of plants and animals, the being of light and colours.[7]

Closely connected with this was the idea of metamorphosis, which gripped König at the beginning of his student years. Through it he came to know the working of creative, formative forces in both nature and in the human being:

> Outside in nature these formative forces work in such a way that they bring all organic forms into being, while inside, in the human soul, they are the creators of our thoughts and ideas.[8]

As he continued to try and understand life forces König stated later:

> In order to grasp life it will be necessary to work on oneself; not only to methodically analyse things outwardly, but awaken in ourselves purified types of imaginations that will then uncover knowledge gleaned from life ... Then we will gain real and scientific knowledge of that which was expressed by the congenial friend of Goethe more than a hundred years ago with the words: 'The body is built up by the spirit'.[9]

In 1921, König encountered the name of Rudolf Steiner for the first time at an exhibition of modern paintings.[10] He came across a triptych that showed Confucius on the left-hand panel, the Buddha on the right-hand panel, and in the centre a picture of a modern worker. Quotations from Confucius and the Buddha had been placed beneath their respective panels and beneath the picture of the worker was a verse by Rudolf Steiner, which described how souls in the dawning new age would feel their connection to the spirit. Although it would be another three years before König began to immerse himself more fully in anthroposophy, nevertheless these lines made a great impression on him:

These words were spoken straight from the heart. But who indeed was this Rudolf Steiner who had been given a place beside the Buddha and Confucius? I obtained one of his books from the university library, *Goethe's World Conception*. Reading this book gave me a sense of deep fulfillment.[11]

What did König read in this book about Goethe?

He was looking for the ideas that live within things, and which make all details of the phenomena appear as if they are growing out of a living wholeness ... [Goethe] wants living concepts by which the spirit of the individual person, according to his individual nature, draws his perceptions together. To know the truth means for him to live in the truth. And to live in the truth is nothing other than, when looking at each individual thing, to watch what inner experience occurs when one stands in front of this thing.[12]

This knowledge and inner experience of music and what is alive permeated the whole of König's life and informed his understanding of music and music therapy.

Anke Weihs, one of the founders of Camphill, and the physician Hans Heinrich Engel were able to experience this. According to Weihs, sitting in meetings with König was like sitting in a chamber orchestra that he was conducting:

At first the theme would sound, then the variations came, the andantes, allegros, and finally the ultimate musical statement ... There was never anything perfunctory, nominal, in any meeting chaired by Dr König. His intuitive knowing how far to go, when to stop a discussion was basically musical. I often had occasion to think of his lectures as sonatas, so musically were they built up.[13]

Engel, who moved to Camphill in 1950 and later collaborated in a decisive way towards the development of music therapy, felt that he had found his teacher in Karl König:

> Here was someone whose words sounded alive, whose thoughts were not shadows, but full of life and truth, whose daily life was filled with the practice of what he demanded of others. Here was truth.[14]

In 1926, König recorded the following inner musical experience in his notebook after a Bruckner Symphony:

> While listening to Bruckner's symphony I realised for the first time (this is how unmusical I had been until then) that the tones are a world in themselves – like a plan that has been pushed into the formed-out physical world and which we do not so easily recognise. Only by paying the greatest attention and by forgetting oneself does one become conscious of it. A new realm is revealed with its own distinctive laws. In how many realms do we live? In as many as we have senses, or bodies and bodily principles? These realms overlap and we are only able to distinguish them with pure concentration.
>
> In psychiatry one also speaks about states of semi-consciousness. Those who are 'ill' describe how suddenly their surroundings become alien to them, 'like fairy land', somebody said today. This means that they wake up in a different realm, such as a sub-physical or a super-physical realm perhaps. But it is also how other 'normal' people can also suddenly become conscious and everything that used to be normal seems like a dream.[15]

In the summer of 1954, König gave a series of lectures called *The Human Soul* in which he attempted to let the soul 'speak of itself'.[16] König describes the landscape of the soul in images, as it is not possible to get to it more closely with methods of natural science. As is the case with the soul, the effect of music cannot be measured or weighed. König makes frequent comparisons between the soul and music that show how far for him they belong together.

> The soul, which in itself is tone and music ...
> The soul, which consists of sound and music ...
> The sense of hearing opens up the world of the soul around us ...

A short passage from *The Human Soul* demonstrates König's image-filled language when describing the soul:

> The soul itself of things and beings begins to speak to us by means of sound and voice and tone. We perceive the mood and the feeling, the longing and the passions of human beings and beasts around us. The rushing wind and the creaking door, the sighing wood and the crackling fire, the moaning and groaning of animals and the speech and song of people reveal the innermost nature of those who sound.
>
> Their soul itself is sound and tone, is song and melody, and we listen from soul to soul when we hear. Whether it is the sound of nature or human speech; whether it is the murmur of water or the tone of a flute; it is soul that is revealed through sound.
>
> Sound is the all-embracing, all-pervading expression of the individual as well as the universal soul. Thus the ear does not reveal the nature of substance as do the senses of smell, taste, sight and warmth. Sound reveals what is

behind the substance, that which permeates the substance with mind and consciousness, with feeling and willing.[17]

In a diary entry, also from the year 1954, König describes how music reveals to him secrets of the art of lecturing:

> Afterwards I prepared myself for the evening lecture and gradually everything grows and flows together what I want to say. However, with this I suddenly experience something completely new to me: it is as though music flowed around me and the rhythm of the lecture sounds through the flow as if a symphony was unfolding itself, or a sonata in four movements. And it feels as though every lecture should be composed of four parts in order to be correct; that is one of the secrets of the art of lecturing.[18]

And at the end of his notes to the lecture 'The Archetypes of the Instruments',[19] given on April 30, 1958, it says:

> What is music? What does it reveal?
> What is expressed and where does it come from?
> From the beginning of humanity it has been the angel of humankind.
> Yet, the totality of the angelic world is the Holy Spirit.
> Music is the body of the Holy Spirit.

In König's notes to the lecture given in Innsbruck on May 5, 1959, to the Society for Physicians he writes what for him is the essence of his remarks:

> This is exactly my intention. I certainly do not intend to present to you theoretical or even ideological analyses, but rather phenomena the interpretation of which poses a challenge to our medical and scientific conscience.[20]

König's lecture notes are visible evidence of the formative musical forces with which he planned his contributions. As for the content, not only the scientific statements, but also the recognition of phenomenology, inner experiences, living concepts and the truth were important to him.

From Vienna to Scotland

König's first proper encounter with anthroposophy took place in 1924 when he was twenty-two years old:

> Following a lecture at the university on the metamorphosis of bones given by Eugen Kolisko[21] (who later became a friend), I came across the book *The Philosophy of Freedom* by Rudolf Steiner ... Here I could read – often in the same words – what I myself had written about the creative forces in nature and human thinking! This was a deep and terrible shock for me. Had I somehow copied it all? Or was it a truth revealed to every searching thinker? My path into anthroposophy now opened up before me and I began to read Rudolf Steiner's seminal works.[22]

For König, the way in which Goethe saw phenomena and the way they were described in the first book he read by Steiner, are for him the starting point for all therapeutic thinking and action.

In 1927 Karl König graduated as a Doctor of Medicine. In October of that same year Ita Wegman came to Vienna. She had been Rudolf Steiner's closest co-worker and had founded the Clinical Therapeutic Institute in Arlesheim near Basel (known as the Ita Wegman Institute from 1971). She asked König if he would be her assistant and, after some hesitation, he accepted the offer. He started at the clinic as well as at the Sonnenhof, where the work in curative education took place.

He came to the Sonnenhof one Sunday in Advent and was shown the Advent Garden. The children gathered there each had an apple with a candle fixed in it and, accompanied by music and singing, they walked around in a spiral that had been laid out with moss. At the centre of the moss spiral was a burning candle from which the children proceeded to light their own candles before walking out of the spiral.

> And suddenly I knew: Yes, this is my future task! To awaken in each one of these children their own spirit light which would lead them to their humanity.[23]

At that time Edmund Pracht worked at the Sonnenhof as a musician. In 1926, he designed a new instrument to be used in eurythmy sessions and the musical work he did with the children. He was dissatisfied with the piano and wanted an instrument that made more musical sounds. While considering what could be taken away from the piano to make it easily accessible to the children, Pracht found that only the frame and the strings were needed. With these considerations in mind he drafted designs that he then discussed with the sculptor Lothar Gaertner. On October 6, 1926, the first prototype of the modern lyre came about. The physicians Ita Wegman and Elisabeth Vreede were among the first to hear the new instrument.

König was to forge a long friendship with Edmund Pracht, and Pracht would visit the Camphill community in Scotland and there compose therapeutic music.

A letter by Pracht to Ita Wegman, only recently discovered in the Ita Wegman Archive, relates a conversation held between König and Pracht on January 28, 1928, about scales, intervals, and their relationship to the history of the development of the skeleton and the human organism. In the notes one can read:

> The main developmental steps of the musical scale correspond to the major moments of the development of the human organism.

On the opposite page is the following remark taken from a lecture given by Rudolf Steiner for eurythmists and music teachers on the inner nature of music and the experience of tone:

> The musical experience will become for the human being proof of the existence of God because the 'I' is experienced twice, once as physical, inner 'I', the second time as spiritual, outer 'I'.[24]

On the same page the phases of embryology have been depicted in drawings made with coloured pencils. It is likely that König and Pracht would have spoken together about this lecture by Steiner. Already in 1928 König must have been working on the connections between the experience of music, music development, embryology and the skeleton. Pracht's accompanying letter to Ita Wegman explains the drawing and adds that at that time there was a study group occupying itself with this theme:

> Dear Dr Wegman,
> Last night I had a conversation with Dr König in which it emerged that the main stages of development of the musical scale correspond to the major moments in the development of the human organism. I made a brief sketch of the content of our conversation on the enclosed page without first adding anything to it at all. It is only on the back of the page that I indicated an explanation

of the most salient points. I wanted to tell you as soon as possible about the ideas relating to this because, as well as the music of the skeleton (music and death), the music of the development of the germ and the embryo (music and life) will also be playing a role in our studies.

With warm greetings,
Your Edmund Pracht

In 1927, the first articles about the experience and the significance of music for the art of healing were published in *Natura*, the magazine edited by Ita Wegman. The authors were Dr H. Walter, Dr Julia Bort, Edmund Pracht, Lothar Gaertner and Eugen Kolisko. One can assume that König was aware of this. That same year König gave the lecture 'On Seeing and Hearing' (a record of this is contained in this book) in which he approached the processes of these senses and their morphology in relation to their polar opposite qualities.

In 1928 König was asked to come to Silesia where his future wife, Tilla, ran a small children's home together with Albrecht Strohschein. While he was in Pilgramshain, König gave lectures and saw a large number of patients.

In 1936 the political circumstances no longer allowed Dr König to live in Germany and so he moved with his family to Vienna. After his escape to Switzerland in 1938 he was able, with Ita Wegman's help, to find a new place to live where he was able to start his work . From 1940 onwards it would continue at the Camphill Estate in Scotland.

The path to music therapy

Music played an important part in the building up of the Camphill movement.[25] König often played the piano and conducted a small Camphill orchestra. For instance, we know that in 1944, during the memorial event for a child who had died, he played parts of Lohengrin and Parzifal, and that he also often played piano for four hands together with Susanne Lissau (later Müller-Wiedemann). In his diary entry of July 15, 1953, he wrote:

> The Hebrides Overture resounds in ancient beauty as do Schubert's Unfinished and his immortal Quintet. It is good to be allowed to live with these sounds and harmonies again.

In those first few years, König invited several musicians to Camphill to make music with the children, among them were Hans Schauder and Ferdinand Rauter.

Hans Schauder met König when Schauder was still a medical student. Through school friends Rudi Lissau and Alex Baum he joined the Youth Group that had formed around König after the latter had left Germany in 1936 and settled again in Vienna. Together with König, Schauder became part of the group of Camphill founders in Scotland in 1939.[26] Schauder was unable to complete his medical studies in Vienna, but he found an opportunity to finish them in Basel where he wrote his dissertation on music therapy and the healing effect of art, a subject that was especially close to his heart.

It was important to Schauder to approach his patients like an artist. He began with the premise that music possesses a particular affinity with the human being, and he wrote about how the inner structure of music is linked to the inner spiritual structure of the human soul. Although Schauder did not have an opportunity to put his ideas into practice, his thesis supervisor nevertheless found his new art-therapy approach worthy of support. He claimed that it 'finally created a basis for music therapy' and subsequently praised it to the university faculty.[27]

This dissertation is in fact one of the first on the theme of healing through music, and König considered Schauder to be one of his most successful students.[28]

The regular Child Conferences that König later held together with his co-workers in Camphill made a lasting impression on Schauder:

> Getting to know a child with Dr König was a fascinating experience for all those involved ... He lived inwardly with the child. Intuition probably also played a role, but the image of the child was the result of hard work. At such meetings we learned to understand the essence and problems of the child and to develop the therapy on that basis ... König possessed great artistic talent, which helped him to feel his way empathetically into the being of the other person.[29]

Besides his work as a physician, Schauder was mainly active with music in Camphill. He gave music and singing lessons to the children and composed music for the plays and the seasonal celebrations that König wrote, as well as for his own plays. In 1944, Schauder, his wife, Lisl, and other Camphill co-workers founded their own curative education initiative at Garvald near Edinburgh. Later he set up a personal counselling service in Edinburgh.[30]

Ferdinand Rauter studied music in Dresden and had lived in London since 1929. In 1940 he was interned on the Isle of Man, as were all the married male co-workers from Camphill. There he met the musicians Norbert Brainin and Peter Schidlof, and he encouraged them to found what would later become the Amadeus Quartet.

König later visited Rauter in London in connection with The Christian Community. There are a number of entries in his diary in which König records further meetings with him over the next few years. They would discuss music and Rauter would often play for König, usually something from Bach or Beethoven, Schubert or Chopin. König began to feel a strong connection to him.

In 1946, Rauter and his family stayed in Camphill for nine months. He was given the task of composing music for the numerous plays written by König, as was Christof-Andreas Lindenberg from 1950 onwards. König describes Rauter's work in the *Superintendent's Report:*

> A special thing that occurred during the past year in Murtle was the major part that music played in the life of the children. The pianist Dr Ferdinand Rauter and the violinist Mr J. Hess taught and played for the children every day. Every morning and evening Dr Rauter played some parts from J.S. Bach's '48 Preludes and Fugues' to the children and teachers. These performances had a beneficial influence on the entire course of the day.[31]

Rauter's daughter, who was born in Camphill, writes about this:

> It seems to be the case that during his time in Camphill my father developed his own music therapy. He later worked with Juliette Alvin, but was disappointed in this, after which he felt more drawn to the School of Nordoff and Robbins.[32]

Rauter worked in Britain as a professional musician. He supported young musicians through the Richard Tauber Prize for young singers and apart from founding the well-known Amadeus Quartet he also founded the Anglo-Austrian Music Society. Moreover, there is an annual 'Ferdinand Rauter Memorial Prize for Accompanists'.

At Whitsun, in 1934, a major conference took place at Pilgramshain in Silesia, with Dr König, Dr Eugen Kolisko, Valborg Werbeck-Svärdström and Dr Karl Schubert. Konig gave the opening lecture, 'Word, Singing and Speaking as Revelation of the Soul', a transcript of which is included in this book. Straight after the conference, Eugen Kolisko held eight lectures on the basic principles of singing therapy for the students of Valborg Werbeck-Svärdström. In the first lecture he spoke about the ear and the sense of hearing and their connection with the larynx:

> Hearing analyses in pure experiences of time,
> development and movement. One could also call
> the activity of our ear an inner conversation between
> dynamic and static in that it spreads its movement over
> the entire body and then makes it come to rest, thus
> conveying the tone to us.[33]

Kolisko was of the opinion that singing as an art and singing as a therapy should not be mixed up:

> If you want to create artistically, you have to have
> loosened and freed up all ties to the organs in such a
> way that you can surrender to the pure formative will as
> if floating freely above the organic. But if you want to
> heal, you first have to bring along a lot of things from the
> organisation. So it's right to realise that you first have to
> heal yourself, so to speak ... As soon as the human being
> is no longer bound or inhibited by his organs,
> then the art emerges in which the human being can
> develop freely.[34]

The time in Pilgramshain occurs in the middle of König's life, as he himself recorded in a biographical sketch from 1939. Did the impetus to research the therapeutic possibilities of language, song, movement and music stem from this time? Music and its therapeutic possibilities have always played an important part in the life of the Camphill community, which was emerging in Scotland from 1939 onwards.

Susanne Lissau's arrival in Camphill on February 1, 1948, marked the beginning of a special period for the development of new therapies. In the *Superintendent's Report 1947–49*, König writes that Lissau, a musician and eurythmist, was dedicating her great and ingenious gifts to children after training in Switzerland for ten years. Her work represented a major part of the curative education offered at Camphill.[35] Together with several therapists she worked intensively on the therapeutic possibilities of music and movement for twelve years, developing various group therapies for children who were deaf or hard of hearing. Various articles appeared on this theme,[36] and in a number of lectures and seminars König, as well as Susanne and her now husband, Dr Hans Müller-Wiedemann, researched this theme more thoroughly, always basing their research on concrete experiences with children.[37] The lecture series that König gave, entitled 'Music and Musical Experience', and his article in the anthology *Musik in der Medizin* [Music in Medicine],[38] really form the high point from this time. From the 1970s onwards, Susanne Müller-Wiedemann taught in the Free Music School, which travelled around schools, and in 1983 she set up training in Curative Eurythmy in Curative Education at the Camphill School Brachenreuthe by the Lake of Constance.

Christof-Andreas Lindenberg moved to Camphill in 1950 and on his first day there gave up his beloved piano for the lyre. He devoted himself to music in the life of the community and especially to music therapy. He wrote many special songs for the seasons, which are still being sung today, and not only in Camphill communities. He was the one who received Paul Nordoff and Clive Robbins in Camphill, when they wanted to get to know the therapeutic possibilities of music in different institutions for curative education in Europe. A number of students of the Free Music School visited Camphill in order to gain experience in music therapy with him. In 1982 Lindenberg moved to America where he devoted much of his time to promoting the lyre and where he also founded the Dorion School for Music Therapy, which he directed for several years. He also regularly visited Berlin to teach at the Center for Music Therapy (Musiktherapeutische Arbeitsstätte), which was founded by Maria Schüppel.

In 1951 the first extended doctors' conference took place in Camphill. König reported there on his first practical research results in the diagnosis and treatment of blind children, children with impaired hearing, with impaired movement and with post-encephalitis.[39] During this workshop Michael Wilson spoke about therapy with coloured shadows, which he was doing with the children in Sunfield Children's Home in Clent, even before this therapy was introduced in Camphill in Scotland.[40]

From 1982 to 1983 I was part of the so-called music department at Murtle Estate. The therapy with coloured shadows was done for a number of children in the *Orpheus Room,* the music therapy room. A calming, relaxing effect, which deepened the breath but also stimulated the will could be observed in the children.

The implementation of this therapy depends on a group of people who work well together and comprises music therapists and eurythmists. Again and again I come across people who manage to fulfil these conditions as well as those of space and technique, thus offering the children a

25

Muskel - Atrophien
mit Glocken spielen heilen.
So auch spastische Lähmungen.
Wo Schicksal gefroren ist,
kann das Gewissen (Glocke)
Weckend wirken.

———

Glockenspiele müssen dauernd
als Zeit - Zeichen einwirken.

———

So wird in Kindern das Gewissen
erwachen.

Healing muscle atrophies
with chime of bells.
Also spasticity.
Where destiny is frozen,
conscience (bell)
can cause awakening.

———

Bells must continually
take influence as "time-markers" ["Zeit-Zeichen"]

———

Thus conscience can awaken in children.

From Karl König's notebook 1951

very special therapy. In a time in which the material aspect of healing is in the foreground these are sources of hope for a therapy that appeals to the whole human being.

In 1952 Karl König asked the professional singer Veronika Bay to come to Camphill to work with deaf and speech-impaired children. Here she had her first experiences in curative education and she developed 'speech-singing' for children whose impulse to speak needed to be stimulated. In 1961 she went to the Netherlands to support her sister and her brother-in-law in establishing Camphill Community Christophorus. Under Hans Heinrich Engel's direction their music therapeutic practice flourished. In addition to that, an international group of people were actively involved in research and work on music-therapy themes as well as on the link between anthroposophical anthropology and the elements of music. In an article in 1974, Veronika Bay described what was essential to her in music therapy:

> With the spiritual individuality of each child in mind
> we try and offer the possibility for the development
> of the individuality, starting from a general approach
> not directed by symptoms. This seems to us a special
> characteristic of the therapeutic work and makes music
> therapy into a profession in its own right.[41]

Veronika Bay occupied herself throughout her life with the qualities of the individual tone and its relationship to the human being. She also worked with the mirrored planetary scales which were developed by Anny von Lange. Veronika Bay taught music therapy in the Netherlands as well as in Germany.

> Her life was devoted to the spirit and to love.
> Through music and music therapy and in the life

of the community she consciously strove for higher developmental aims. Anthroposophy was her inspiration in life and she offered its fruits to her fellow human beings until her old age.[42]

In the meeting of music therapists in Camphill in 1961 and 1962, work was done in relation to the 'life processes' described by Rudolf Steiner in his lecture series *The Riddle of Humanity*. In January 1961, König gave three lectures about music, which unfortunately were not recorded. König's notes of the discussions in 1962, which were written down afterwards, can be found in the chapter 'Music Therapy Conferences' in this volume.

The therapeutic impulse in the curative education movement remained very close to König's heart, and in 1963 he helped to establish a college in Camphill dedicated to the many therapies and treatments that had been developed in the Camphill movement, including music therapy.

During the last year of his life König was still exploring ideas relating to the musical form of the life processes. As a result of König's encounter with the musical scientist Hermann Pfrogner, research into the development of music therapy started at Camphill Community Christophorus in the Netherlands in the early 1960's but came to a premature end with the sudden death of Engel in 1973. After his work with Anny von Lange, Pfrogner had been occupied with the inner movements in relation to the intervals and had come across results that made König enthusiastic.[43] Afterwards, König asked Pfrogner to occupy himself with the life processes as well. Correspondence between König and Pfrogner about these birth processes of music therapy is contained in this volume. This also relates to plans for training in music therapy and art therapy in Perceval. In a letter of June 18, 1965, Hermann Pfrogner called König the 'spiritual patron of a reality-based music therapy which can be taught and learned'.

Lectures by Hans Heinrich Engel on the outcomes of this research work in which music therapists and eurythmists from Ireland, Scotland, the Netherlands, Switzerland and Germany also took part and which he conducted in Ireland, Switzerland and in Berlin, were published in 1999 (and in English in 2013).[44] From König's attempts to come closer to the relationship between spiritual science, music and physiology, a music therapy had emerged based on Goethean phenomenology and anthroposophical spiritual science, the healing effect of which many children and adults were allowed to experience, now no longer only in the Camphill schools and communities for adults with special educational needs.

On the documents in this volume

1. Articles by Karl König

It is easy to get a general overview of the number of published articles by König on music therapy. Almost all of them appeared between 1952 and 1958 and relate mainly to the work König did with children in Camphill who had hearing impairments.

In 1952 König wrote an article for *Beiträge zur Erweiterung der Heilkunst* [Contributions to the Furtherance of the Art of Healing] called 'Deafness in Children: The Ability to Hear and Tumour Formation'. It is addressed to a wider audience of physicians and in it he refers to two quotations from Rudolf Steiner's first course to doctors: 'As early as childhood, the congenitally deaf would have been predisposed to the worst sort of tumour formation if they had not been born deaf',[45] and: 'The ear is an internal tumour in the human being, but kept within normal limits'.[46] The article contains an extensive report on research König carried out with nine deaf children using Dr Ehrenfried Pfeiffer's crystallisation method. König gave a vivid description of the music therapy with deaf children in the *Superintendent's Report* of the year 1955. An article written for the English journal *Spastics Quarterly* at Christmas 1954 and published at Easter 1955 in *Das Seelenpflegebedürftige Kind* [The Child in Need of Spiritual Care], describes the use of coloured shadows with musical accompaniment in therapy for children with paralysis. Excerpts from this article are included in 'Therapy with Music and Coloured Shadows'.[47]

In 1955 König also wrote an article about the lyre, included in this volume, in which he reviewed a book by Edmund Pracht on lyre playing. König quotes from the book:

> When practising and playing the lyre one senses the mystery which also today lies within the musical tone, and one feels called upon to search for one's spiritual sources.[48]

The most well-known article by König on music therapy is 'Music Therapy in Curative Education', which he wrote at the request of Hildebrand Richard Teirich for inclusion in the book *Musik in der Medizin* in 1957. Teirich wanted to report on the correlation between the effects of music on patients in relation to their pathology, and to draw attention to methods that had already proved helpful in psychotherapy. König was one of the sixteen authors approached by Teirich, with Teirich asking König to write from an anthroposophical point of view. The book appeared in 1958 and was the first book about music therapy in Europe; a similar book had already been published in America in 1948 called *Music and Medicine* by Dorothy M. Schullian and Max Schoen.

In the article König describes his experiences with music therapy in curative education. He mentions his precursors in this field, whom he considered to be important and upon whose results he based his work, going all the way back to the nineteenth-century pioneer in curative education Edouard Séguin. The closing section of the article provides a schematic sketch of the landscape of music therapy in which there is a description of how König continued to develop the relationship between music and the human being as described in Rudolf Steiner's *The Inner Nature of Music and the Experience of Tone*.

König stresses the importance in music therapy of not just playing music or of 'playing what one feels like' for the patient:

> With regard to a newly formulated music therapy we have to try first of all to analyse music as to its archetypal elements, and then to explore these elements in their effect on the human being. When these first steps are accomplished, then a general, as well as a specific music therapy can be developed, for instance in the field of curative education.[49]

A review of the book by Gisbert Huseman was published in 1959 stating that art as therapy has as its mission to keep the human being on the right path between the clutches of matter and the loss of self.[50] He sees these dangers in various directions in music therapy. He welcomes König's article, 'Music Therapy in Curative Education', in which a summary is given of the method according to which he and other curative teachers had already been working with music therapy for a long time. Husemann writes that art in its various guises should again be introduced into the activity of physicians. Finally, he expresses the hope that these steps would remain in the realm of the laws of art and not be subjected to the laws of mainstream medical science.

It is worth noting that after the publication of *Musik in der Medizin* two music therapy societies were founded, one in Vienna[51] and one in London.[52] The music therapist Alfred Schmölz[53] clearly traced the founding of the Austrian society for the promotion of music therapy in 1958 and the training for music therapy in 1959 back to Teirich and the publication of *Musik in der Medizin*. A symposium with the same name was held in Velden am Wörthersee in 1959.[54] König was invited by Teirich, but he was unable to attend.[55]

Musik in der Medizin reached many people who at that time were involved in music therapy and König's contribution is still mentioned in scientific writings to this day.

König intended to write a book about hearing and movement, and several articles, some of which had already been published in *Die Drei,* are linked to this. One article that has been included in this volume, and which was most likely written in 1963, is 'The Four Stages of Hearing'. In it, König differentiates between noise, sound, speech sound and tone, something that resounds again and again in the lectures he gave to music therapists in 1958 as well as in his lectures about the senses.[56]

2. Transcripts of lectures

Music and its relationship to the human being permeates a large part of these lectures given by König.

In the lecture 'On Seeing and Hearing' from 1927, König describes the functions of the eye and the ear and brings them into connection with the microcosmic human being and the macrocosm.

In the lecture given in Pilgrimshain on the 'The Word,

Singing and Speaking as Revelation of the Soul', König turns to the process of how speech originated:

> In our time language has merely become what is called 'naming', but it used to be a living creative force which was working in a formative way in the whole world.

In 1958 König gave various lectures on the theme of music and music therapy. Included in this volume are 'Musical Instruments', three lectures he gave under the title of 'Music and Musical Experience', and 'Music in Curative Education'. In his notes for the lectures on music and musical experience, König mentions that there were different reasons why music should be discussed precisely in our time:

1. The need to write something about music and curative education. This made me aware of how incomplete and insufficient music therapy is that is being practised in the world at present.
2. Yet, at the same time, I was also able to experience how completely insufficient our own attempts are that we have so far undertaken.

König here refers to the article he wrote for *Musik in der Medizin*, as well as to the other articles published in it. As is clear from the above quote, he was happy neither with the way music therapy was being practised more broadly in the world, nor with his own particular efforts. This might be the reason why in his lifetime very little was published by him on music therapy and why his articles have not been published until now. What König had worked on for his articles must now also be heard by the co-workers in Camphill. As he had done in 1934 in Pilgramshain, König again spoke about musical instruments and music at Whitsun, because he was conscious of the relationship between music and Whitsun.

3. Letters

The correspondence between Karl König and Hildebrand Richard Teirich that accompanied the publication of the book *Musik in der Medizin* has been included in this volume.

In January of both 1961 and 1962 discussions and workshops about music were held in Scotland. In the notes of January 6, 1962, which König put together following that year's discussions, he called this research work a musical physiology.

> Thus a first beginning of a musical physiology has come about. This is linked with Eugen Kolisko, whom we remembered at the end of the course.

The correspondence between Karl König and the musical scientist Hermann Pfrogner gives some insight into how this research work with the music therapists and the physician Dr Hans Heinrich Engel in the Netherlands proceeded.

4. Karl König's lecture notes

The choice we have made in relation to the lecture notes shows the different ways König devoted himself to this theme over time.

The two lectures given in London in 1943 under the title 'On the Ear and Hearing', deal with how the ear and hearing evolved in humans out of the different ways in which animals hear. The second lecture describes how language, too, comes about in the course of evolution.

In 'A Study on Hearing', given in 1953, König develops the theme of metamorphosis in relation to hearing and speaking. This theme then resounds again in the lecture he gave to physicians, also in 1953, called 'Movement of the Limbs and Cancer Prophylaxis'. This goes into the connection between hearing, the movement of the limbs and cancer, something König had reported on in great detail the year before in the lecture 'About the Treatment of Sensory Disorders in Children'.

In 1958 König gave the three lectures on music and musical experience mentioned above. These lectures are especially important because König considers the therapeutic effect of music. Nevertheless, it is only with third of the three lectures, given on June 18, that a possible therapeutic application is hinted at. There are no prescriptions, but König refers the reader to their own experience in the anthropological-musical context. It is in this light that all his lecture notes and studies should be seen, as he himself searches for these contexts and stimulates people to think for themselves.

In 1960, in Brachenreuthe, König gave the lecture 'Movement and Hearing'. Here he stated that for many years it had been one of his closest concerns to gain a deeper understanding of hearing and movement, of the unique structure of the ear and of the world of movement:

> Looking into it more closely we find that we are not dealing with isolated phenomena in either, but with processes connected with the totality of our structure, of the body, the soul and the spirit.

In 1960 König gave a lecture to physicians about the kidney and the ear, in which he researched the intimate link between the two organs:

Above in the ear there is hearing, down below in the kidneys, music is made.

König's notes of this lecture, 'About the Kidney and Hearing', are also included in this volume.

5. Sketches by Karl König

The hand-drawn illustrations included in this book are either taken directly from König's notebooks or are modified versions of sketches König drew.

Coda

Speaking from a musical-anthropological point of view, a development took place in Karl König's endeavours in music therapy that led from seed to the new human being, from the prime to the octave. The seed, the prime, was König's first musical impulse, which then developed via the second, his occupation with what is living, to the third and fourth when the research into the healing elements of music began. The fifth was reached when gradually more people gathered around König who were actively taking up his impulses towards healing. The sixth and the seventh bring the development outwards through lectures, articles and conferences. Yet when the octave had been reached something new began. The seeds of music therapy that had been laid in the hearts of many people began to grow and bear fruit when König crossed the threshold into the spiritual world in 1966.

Lectures and Articles

The Word, Singing and Speaking as Revelation of the Soul

Lecture given in Pilgramshain, May 19, 1934

It is fitting today, on the eve of the Whitsun Festival, for us to say something about the essential being of the Word. The festivals are times when the Word, the resurrecting Word, is ever and again celebrated as it lives in nature. Whitsun is just one of those festivals during which we can speak particularly and most profoundly about the nature of speaking and singing and what they represent for the world and human beings. The fact that it is possible to speak about such things is down to what Rudolf Steiner has communicated to us through anthroposophy, which is an all-embracing understanding of the Word as a living being that works in us and in nature. In order to speak about the Word and gain insight into the most varied regions of existence, we have to approach it from many different sides, more so than is usual when we ordinarily look at how human beings stand in relation to nature.

If we visit one of our modern museums and allow what has been gathered there from the various cultures to impress itself upon us, not only of works of art but also handcrafted objects from daily life, then one might be able to experience something of the development of the human soul over the course of millennia. In an enormous room in the Pergamon Museum in Berlin the so-called Ishtar Gate has been set up. This formed part of one of the larger gates that led into the inner city of Babylon and was built in the sixth century bc at the command of King Nebuchadnezzar II. It has been reconstructed with part of the Processional Way, a walled approach that led from the Ishtar Gate to the Euphrates. The bricks that formed the walls of this wide corridor carried reliefs of lions and the Persian gods, including the goddess Ishtar.

Walking along the passage that leads to the gate, you see the lions standing open-jawed on either side, as though waiting to devour you. You must proceed, upright, in order to enter the temple through that portal. From this you can get a glimpse of how the human beings of that time felt themselves to be embedded in a network of relationships that included truly mythological figures, and how this whole background finds expression in such a work of art. Everything that was experienced as being the background of natural existence, has expressed itself in this great work of art, and you can feel how human beings had to go through this passage, looking neither left nor right, without allowing anything from this background to approach them and potentially overwhelm them.

Then you go up the steps to the Pergamon Altar, this marvellous clear form with the delicate pillars. You can imagine people clad in white, standing on these temple steps talking, and yet you are also surrounded by nature, everything that is happening there is nature: the clouds, the blue sky – everything participates.

Later on, you might come upon one of the pictures of the Madonna by Raphael in such a museum. There you see a complete transformation of the human soul. The mother of God is sitting with the child on her lap. In the background the landscape becomes bright, and you could almost feel that some angelic being might still peer through. But the background has been done in perspective; human beings no longer take an active part in nature: the natural world has become no more than a backdrop. What was alive in the pictures of these painters some four or five hundred years ago has been lost even more in today's consciousness. Not only has nature become a backdrop, but it has almost vanished completely; it has become silent and can no longer speak. We no longer understand the wind, the passing clouds or the twinkle of the stars. We stand as beings outside of time and space, estranged from nature. One can see expressed in this image the mysterious weaving between nature and the human soul that human beings have always endeavoured to grasp.

The human soul has its own connection to nature, be it conscious or unconscious, and with it we participate in what happens around us. One clear example is the change from night to day. Although we have emancipated ourselves from this transition to a certain extent (we no longer have to go to sleep just because the sun has set), we are still affected by this inborn rhythm of sleeping and waking. It was Rudolf Steiner who pointed out that human beings stand in an inverse connection to this natural rhythm: when we lie down to sleep our soul-spiritual entity leaves our body and shines over our sleeping form as the sun shines over the earth by day; when we awaken, then this soul-spirit-sun withdraws into our body just as the sun sets in the evening and disappears behind the earth. If we keep this image in mind, of the sun rising in the morning and setting in the evening, it becomes possible to clarify the relationship between the soul and body for our consciousness.

Now we might ask ourselves, how is it that we are able to speak?

An enormous amount of thought has been given to language. There are whole libraries of books about the origin of human speech. And yet it remains a mystery how one should imagine the way in which speech originated. Particularly in the last years of the nineteenth century much has been written about this, but even at the present time science has not gone beyond what was published then. It is amazing the primitive way in which the origins of language has been spoken about. For instance, one theory imagined that early human beings, who had only taken the first steps away from being apes, became attentive to the world around them and began to name things: first a flower, then a tree. In any case one had the idea that in some sort of way things were named arbitrarily. Then, in addition, they began to express the emotions they had within them.

But all of this is something that has been imposed upon the human soul. It is not something the soul could ever have done, because it has never possessed the capacity to do it. Just as each animal and each plant has its own inherent laws, which means that one cannot develop out of the other, so too the human soul has its own laws according to which it develops. It could never have happened that a human soul stepped out into the world and then began to express itself in speech, because the human soul does not function like that. If one really studies how language came about, and this can be found in the work of Rudolf Steiner, then one finds out that human beings first began to sing.[1] That was first, not speaking. Only gradually, over the course of human evolution, did a recitative element emerge in which the rhythms and delivery of ordinary speech developed. It was from this that what we call language arose.

Nowadays, language is dead, but once upon a time it was alive. It was a creative power, able to work within the creative processes of the world. Human beings could encourage plants to grow and create forms out of the earth through the power of their singing. They could enchant others through words, capturing and destroying other souls through language. Human beings have forgotten this because language has died, though it was necessary that this happened.

Today language has become more or less what you might call descriptive, denotative. We are no longer able to affect the world with language in a formative way.

But how did language come about? We only need to observe how small children bring forth their first sounds, not the yelling or the whimpering of the first months because that is not language. One sees how children after the first year begin to react to their surroundings. The souls of small children are full of wonder and this wonder expresses itself by bringing forth a sound. They say, 'Ah,' for 'Ah' is nothing other than the sound of wonder. The first sound made by humankind was 'Ah', and this was sung, because wonder and speaking are fundamentally the same. When the human soul experiences wonder towards the existence of the world, then speech emerges out of the realm of the soul we bear within us. It is not something created by air in the larynx; it is the child of the soul, born out of wonder as an expression of it. And just as the regions of the earth are different from one another, so was this 'speech' different as it came forth out of the soul in each region.

Not only human beings speak, but also animals speak or emit sounds. Let us look at how the animals send forth their sounds. The plant and the lower animals are silent. Some animals are able to create noise using parts of their anatomy, for example, male crickets that rub their front wings together, but these sounds do not come from within them, they do not express an inner nature. But you only need to listen to the croaking of a frog, the bellowing of the cow, or the neigh of the horse to realise that these sounds are like the animal itself. A croaking sound is as watery and spongy as the animal that croaks; the noise the cow makes is so intimately bound up with the beast that it is unable to sound other than it does. One should really be able to discern from the sound an animal makes in this way its whole shape and form of existence; one can grasp its essential nature if one has learned to observe it.

The singing of birds on the other hand is nothing but a noise, but in the most exalted and beautiful sense conceivable. Christian Morgenstern wrote something very beautiful about the singing of birds:

> You little bird in yonder tree, dear bird
> what is your song, your song on earth?
> Your little song is God's own Word,
> Your little throat is God's own mouth.
>
> 'I sing' does not yet sing from you,
> It is the sound of creations might,
> Still pure and in fashion new,
> In you, you small and sweet delight.[2]

Morgenstern expresses it wonderfully: it is not 'I sing' but 'it sings'. The whole divine power of creation sings through this bird, its throat is still the mouth of God. There is a great difference between the singing of a human being and the sound of an animal, for in the sounding of an animal the supersensible nature of music is revealed that lives and works in the natural world, the power of sound that dwells in all things.

Rudolf Steiner once described the way people celebrated festivals in earlier times. At the time of St John's festival, under the guidance of their priests, people came together to prepare themselves. They formed choirs and chanted certain songs whilst moving to the sounds. They sensed in the singing and rhythmical pacing during the night of the festival something arising in the world that was still in the hands of the Gods, and which human beings were allowed to see only once a year. Their singing streamed upwards and after their singing they waited in stillness for the gods to answer. When wonder is freed up it becomes a question. We can feel something of a questioning quality arising in our soul when we sing and speak. But when we speak we must also learn to hold back, for only if we listen will we hear the answer to our question. The speaking human being is really only a human being when they begin to listen. Once a year, in earlier times, people moved and sang rhythmically, then waited for the gods to answer. And their own 'I-Being' appeared to them.[3]

Rudolf Steiner said that even when we hear the birds singing outside, the larks and the nightingales, this singing is not only for their enjoyment, it is necessary for the whole of nature. For with that singing something rises up that reaches a certain boundary of our terrestrial sphere, and divine powers then descend to the earth with the song and give forming, creative forces to the animal kingdom. Birdsong becomes a garment for the powers of the gods.[4]

Following in the mood of this description one can penetrate further into the essentials of singing and speaking. Singing and speaking can be seen as children of the soul that emerges from it when wonder becomes a question. Just as we inhale and exhale, so also speech is a breathing process of question and answer. Speaking and questioning, speaking and answering, are processes that belong together. Asking is speaking and answering is also speaking. Between asking and answering there is the realm of listening. We must keep this trinity in mind if we wish to define more closely speech and singing: the question is the first part, listening is the second, and answering the third. Even the fact that we can question and answer each other has developed because we ourselves have become able to give birth to speech out of our own soul.

Plato, in one of his wonderful dialogues known as the Crito, pointed out that it can be by no means possible that the naming of things arose from purely arbitrary impulses of the human soul; rather the name and what is named are intimately connected. Plato leads his pupils to understand that the name is nothing other than the inner aspect of the thing itself. If I say 'tree', it is not merely an outer description, instead this very being reveals its most inward form. If I say 'cloud', then the inner nature of the cloud reveals itself in my soul. Human beings can give names to the beings of nature because the soul has, to a certain degree, become a vessel in which nature can express its innermost aspect, and this most inward aspect *is the name* of what human beings speak the name of.

If I say 'tree', then I say to it: 'that is you'. My speech is name-giving. It is nothing other than an answer to the mysterious questions that arise from the primal ground of all existence and are embedded in the garment of nature, in everything that is physical and expresses itself in form and in colour. The human being calls them by their name and thereby their most inward nature reveals itself. It used to be so that one could feel, 'When I speak the name of a thing, I have power over it'. One really has something of the inmost essential being of a thing if one can call it by name. In this way human beings, by beginning to question, beginning to listen and thus receiving an answer, become themselves the answer to the otherwise unrevealed questions of nature.

To come a little closer to the secret of speaking and singing, one might consider the following consideration. How is it possible for us to speak at all? Even in today's natural science one knows nothing about speaking. We know that there is a larynx, this remarkable formation that is connected to the air-passages and so on, but if one asks what speech really is, one can only say that it is something like rhythmical vibrations brought about in the air. For the breathing flow of air passes into the larynx and this causes the air to vibrate rhythmically: the air is shaped and the sound is formed. But the air has as much to do with speaking as the earth does with the human being, which is to say that if one were to say that the earth *is* the human being, then it would be the same as saying that the air is speech. Of course, we need the earth to walk around, and in the same fashion we need the air in order to speak. Air is the ground on which the tone lives. We have to form the air rhythmically, but with that we form the garment, the body of the tone.

We need to look at speaking as it works through the whole human being, as it develops out of the threefold nature of the human being. Just as we carry our thinking in our head, and in our limbs we bear our will, and the two must work together, true speech can only be formed when it is rooted in the will and in the clarity of our thinking. Only when we can think and activate our will can we form speech properly, because only then can directed thought be spoken out. Our feeling then becomes the necessary garment. We really have to consider the human being as a whole, and how thinking, feeling and the willing need to work in clarity and harmony, to realise how out of this trinity speaking and singing is formed.

We have already described how the human soul can be understood using an image of sleeping and waking. It is with waking up that the soul can continue its work within us, and with this submerging of the human soul into corporeality language can also come about. Proper speech is present when soul and spirit have entered the earthly body.

When the sun sets the stars appear and the heavens reveal their magnificence. When the soul-spirit-sun of our being sets in the earthly body, then also a starry sky is born: namely, speech. Speech is nothing other than an image of the heavens we see at night: in the vowels we find expressed the forces of the planets, and in the consonants the forces of the fixed stars. Everything that appears to us at night is present when we are awake and speak. In this way speaking is the revelation of the heavens that we behold each night.

Through this we can experience how the human soul becomes an endless realm in itself, one that is an image of all that surrounds us in nature. We consider our thoughts and concepts and find them in the animals around us. We consider our will and see it as cosmic will, frozen into the world of stones and crystals. We look at our feeling from the nightside of the soul and recognise it as the world of plants. Just as outside we have wind and weather, lightning and thunder, passing clouds, gleaming stars, growing plants, stones, plants and animals, in the same way this has also been created within our soul. Our soul is the whole realm of nature as seen from the other side. In our thoughts the inner nature of animal existence is expressed, in our feeling that of the plants, and in our will the mineral world.

Going beyond the faculty of speech, if we want to find an image of the word in nature, then we should study the plant world. The word in our soul and plants in nature form a unity. As individual plants grow they undergo a metamorphosis of root, stalk, leaf, flower and fruit. We can see this in the outer world, and it is but an image of what we speak. The plants grow out of the ground just as our speech emerges out of the nature of our will, and just as plants transform according to the formation of the ground, in the same way speech also transforms according to the individual nature of our will. If you study plants you can find that in them, too, there is an expression of what is revealed when we ask questions and gives answers. Also the element of listening one can find there: The blossom is nothing but question expressed in a natural form. It sends questions out into the cosmos, just as the singing birds send questions forth and as the human being sends out thousands of questions into the world. The question in its natural form is to be found in all the blossoms and flowers. When the blossoms fall then listening arises to which the cosmos gives a response, the response becomes the fruit.

Spring is question, autumn is answer. Formed-out question and formed-out answer meet us there. What is just fixed in the physical, we are able to transform anew from within for we are continuously able to ask and to answer anew. Also the earth expresses itself in the blossom and receives the answer from the heavens through the fruit. Rilke expressed this in his 'Sonnets to Orpheus':

> Spring has again returned. The Earth
> is like a child that knows many poems,
> many, o so many ... For the hardship
> of such long learning she receives the prize.
>
> Strict was her teacher. The white
> in the old man's beard pleases us.
> Now, what to call green, to call blue,
> we dare to ask: she knows, she knows!
>
> Earth, now free, you happy one, play
> with the children. We want to catch you,
> joyful Earth. Only the most joyful can do it.
>
> Oh, what her teacher taught her, such plenitude,
> and that which is pressed into roots and long
> heavy, twisted trunks: she sings, she sings!

Indeed, in winter the whole glory of the stars takes shape in the roots of plants. In this simple way the word can reveal itself within the soul of someone who devoted his whole life to the study of the mysterious connection between nature and the soul.

In this way we can find a true basis for a deeper understanding of the word and speech. There would still be much to say about it, and I also hope to be able to mention a few aspects concerning the differentiation between singing and speaking. If one wants to learn something about singing it would be necessary to grasp the whole of the human being in their fourfold nature: the physical, the etheric or life-forces, the soul element and the spiritual. Everything takes on form in the trinity of thinking, feeling and willing. Then those aspects enter this trinity that speak out of the physical air, out of the life forces, out of the soul quality, out of the nature of the 'I'. The speech we form with our teeth, our jaws and so on, is shaped quite physically. Then something comes into the process that we call tone: it is life itself that is formed out of the flowing of sound. The way in which speech, tone and flowing sound unite, we were also able to see this flowing together in nature by observing the world of plants.[5]

The main thing I wanted to express was something to help guide our understanding towards the all-embracing forces of language. Language has become dead, the word has died, and we need once again to acquire at least an inkling of the forces of language as it once was. If we look into the world, then it can become for us a revelation of singing and speaking. The whole of nature sounds and sings. We conduct our daily life in constant dialogue with our destiny: in all that we do, we are asking, and in all that comes towards us, we find answers. We stand in life in such a way that as human beings we are sending out questions and destiny responds.

Out of this whole interplay of question and answer between human beings and destiny something special comes about. Our larynx, with whose help we are able to speak, is the organ of questioning. As a result of this questioning there arises a second organ, that of listening, the ear. And our head is the answer, it is in fact the response to all that we have done in our life. On a number of occasions Rudolf Steiner described how the head is the outcome of our previous earthly life, it is the transformation of what we once did in life. Out of this interplay between life and destiny, question and answer, our head is formed. You will be aware that with our head everything is formed out in the finest details, which is only partly so for the larynx. That which was merely indicated, as a draft so to speak with the larynx, is formed out to completion with the head. Both have the same basic form, the larynx only indicated, because it is question, blossom, the head formed out because it is fruit, is answer, answer to our past earth life.

As human beings we are the bearer of the word within nature. With this we have received a task. The whole of nature is a question, and if we not only utter the outer name but add to this the inner forces that are at work in the innermost being of nature, then we follow the path that Rudolf Steiner wished to lead us along:

> I once said in my book entitled *A Theory of Knowledge Implicit in Goethe's World Conception*, that living thinking represents the spiritual form of communion among humankind. For as long as we give ourselves up to our mirror-thoughts about external Nature, we do nothing but repeat the past. We live in corpses of the Divine. When we ourselves bring life into our thoughts, then, giving and receiving communion through our own being, we ally ourselves with the element of Divine Spirit which permeates the world and assures its future.[6]

Or, as he expressed it in a quote from Goethe: 'Perception of the idea within the actual is the true communion of the human being'.

If we learn to hear the inner word of nature then we shall reach the true communion, which is to become the answer to the question posed by creation itself. And we shall only be able to give this answer when we hear the word that speaks in everything. If we can hear once again the word that lives and weaves in plants, animals and clouds, not as a mythological figure but as an idea redeemed by the thoroughly Christianised human being, then our own being will be the answer to the questioning and waiting creation. Rudolf Steiner described this path and its goal with the words 'In the Spirit's World-All-Thoughts the soul awakens'.[7] This is the true Whitsun word.

Musical Instruments

Lecture given in Newton Dee, May 25, 1958

Dear Friends,

We have tried throughout the last months to prepare ourselves again this year for the experience of Whitsun. We have tried to go as consciously as possible, as far as we are individually able, through the forty days from Easter to Ascension, and then tried to experience these very important ten days that stretch from Ascension to Whitsun. Now we have arrived, we again stand as it were, in the glory of Whit Sunday. Every year anew – I think I can speak for all of us, dear friends – we learn to see Whitsun not as a festival of our present time only, but more and more as a festival that will find its full weight and complete unfolding in the future of humanity. There, humanity will learn to know that Whitsun is not a festival that can be reached by the modern intellect, but can only be experienced intimately within the centre of the human soul, where the human spirit unfolds itself. The seed of the human spirit is the seed for Whit Sunday.

But, dear friends, when we try to sense our way further – a little bit deeper, a little more thoroughly – into the whole substance of Whitsun, if we do not only remember what it recalls – the tremendous event of the first day of Pentecost when, as it is described in the Acts of the Apostles, the disciples were gathered together in the Upper Room and they heard a mighty rushing wind and saw cloven tongues of fire settling upon the heads of each one of the Twelve – if we do not only recall this and we do not only rejoice in the waking up of nature around us, if we try to enter as I said into the substance of Whitsun – then my dear friends, more and more one has the impression that something very special draws near to the human soul.

If, for instance, you study the pictures from the early and later Middle Ages that tried to describe the event of Whitsun, you have the impression that this subject does not lend itself to painting. Hardly any of the great and famous painters has attempted to present a picture of Whitsun. If it is done in the old illuminations, for example, or in some of the very simple and primitive paintings of the Middle Ages, you have the impression that you stand before an image that indeed bears something in it, but this something is not really expressed in the painting. You see Mary, sitting in the middle, with the Holy Dove descending from above and either side of her, six on one side and six on the other, the disciples: it is something strangely symmetrical that reminds the human soul of an impression, yet it does not *present* this impression as it were. If you ask yourself what this means, you might gradually come to understand that neither in colour nor in form can Whitsun be portrayed. There is only one element whereby the Whitsun element can be expressed, and that is in music. Within the substance of Whitsun, dear friends, there lives the element of sound: be it the spoken word, be it the moving of the spirit through the elements (the wind in this instance), be it the sound of music itself, be it the harmony of the cosmos – Whitsun is a festival that can only be approached if we gradually learn to live within the world of sound and music. And these paintings that I have described to you, they are nothing other than depictions of musical instruments, musical instruments that appear in human form. And one would have to 'play' these paintings, as it were, to hear what they want to tell us. For this reason, I thought it would be justified if we occupy ourselves tonight with the element of music, especially with musical instruments. This might sound profane to begin with, but perhaps at the end of all that I will say to you tonight, you will think differently, dear friends.

Musical instruments belong to the things that humanity during its development on earth has made. I do not think, dear friends, that there is anything so mysterious, anything so wonderful and at the same time so miraculous, as the forms of musical instruments. All human-made things are of tremendous interest: whether you follow up the history of a chair or a stool or a table or a vase or whatever there is, you can be deeply engrossed and think nothing else is as interesting as this. But among all of these things – these human-made things with their various functions – there are the musical instruments. And perhaps in their form, in their imagery and enormous variety, they are something that can be described in a special way on a day like Whit Sunday. You see, dear friends, scientists who today try to describe the development of musical instruments in the course of human evolution, start with the idea that humanity to begin with was very primitive, and therefore it must have had very simple and very primitive instruments in order to make a little bit of noise (presumably because human beings were like children and so liked things as noisy as possible!). Gradually, as our thinking woke up and we became as intellectual as we are today, we liked things a little bit more complicated. And yet the same scientists who state this must also confess in astonishment that as soon as musical instruments appear they are already very complicated. They explain this away by saying that musical instruments must have existed for thousands of years before, otherwise they could not be as refined and complete as they are. We find, for instance, quite refined instruments in the Sumerian culture and in old Egypt. Instruments which show that music has been one of the great companions of humanity since the beginning of time. But if we go a little further into the past history of humanity, we find instruments that are very different from what we are used to today, or even seven or eight hundred years ago, maybe even a thousand. Speaking now from the point of view of spiritual science because ordinary research does not go back this far, one has the impression that in primeval times the elements of air and light, and the sound or chemical ether, the warmth ether and the life ether were still so much alive, so creative and full of strength, that they formed musical instruments by the hand of human beings. During this time, which I would like to clearly define as the Atlantean epoch and the period immediately after Atlantis, it would not really be true to say that humans being played instruments; rather, a living nature built and formed these instruments and used the human hand in order that they should sound within it.

You will find, for instance, forms made from clay that can quite rightly be described as primitive, clay drums, but they are not large, you could hold them in your hands. You find in the early Celtic period very strange kinds of trumpets, the so-called lures. They are huge instruments usually found in pairs, which suggests that two were to be played together. It is a kind of bell that sits on a long, curving tube with a mouthpiece at the other end (that is at least what one thinks today).

You find all kinds of forms made out of clay that make noise (although probably it is only today that they make noise, once upon a time they produced beautiful sounds). But what forms do these instruments have? They have the form of human beings and various kinds of animals, and you can blow through them or shake them. But one can have the impression that it is not an instrument that human beings consciously use. Rather, it is nature that, in the same way that it forms plants, flowers and animals, forms these instruments and gives them over into the hands of humanity. We need to come to a new understanding of the difference between the instruments of today and those we might consider to be more natural instruments, not yet human instruments.

After this period – after Atlantis had come to an end and humanity spread east and started to form the Post-Atlantean civilisations of India and Persia and so on – from this time onwards three types of instruments accompanied humanity that we still see today: wind instruments, string instruments and percussion instruments, which are beaten like a drum. There is no doubt for me that within this threefoldness of musical instruments we find how the human component of the musical instrument reveals itself. Many of us have come to a certain clarity about this. Through indications Rudolf Steiner has made one usually comes to a first order of these three types of instruments. I can only say 'through indications Rudolf Steiner has made', because they are not as clear as one would like; they are suggestions with which we have to work, and about this we will speak tonight.

One speaks of the wind instruments as belonging to the forces of human thought, the string instruments to the forces of feeling, and the percussion instruments to the forces of will. We could therefore say: thinking and feeling and willing, in the existence of musical instruments, seem to reveal themselves in the form of wind instruments, string instruments and percussion instruments. I try to be as clear as possible when speaking of the 'existence' of musical instruments, meaning also their spiritual reality. This preliminary order of instruments is somewhat simple as it is only a very superficial order. It does not reveal much yet to those who really want to understand the nature of an instrument.

Something else Rudolf Steiner mentioned, and which I think is of much greater importance, is that melody, harmony and rhythm belong to these three types of instruments, although again this is only a hint, an indication.[1] If you study the eurythmy figures that Steiner designed for minor and major and several other musical forms, you will suddenly find that instead of 'melody' he uses the word 'melos', instead of 'harmony' he uses 'rhythm', and instead of 'rhythm' he speaks of 'tact'.[2] Now I do not mean to suggest that Steiner is contradicting himself, not in the least. What I mean is that such indications are prompting us, are trying to teach us: be careful, watch, try to understand and not simply to accept.

Taking this as an indication only and nothing else, we can now ask ourselves, what are wind instruments, and what is the real difference between wind and string instruments? Let us do this first of all, dear friends, simply in a morphological way: let us try to understand the form of a flute or an oboe or a horn in comparison to a string instrument, which is so completely different. Have you ever considered very deliberately the enormous, one could almost say the polarised, difference between a pipe and a violin or a mandolin or a cello? We can start from a simple observation and ask, what is the difference? Why is the one formed like this and the other like that, and what is aroused in us when we hear a pipe or a flute or an oboe or a horn play? Try and recall these very different sounds. Think also of the deep sounds of the harp or the high sounds of a fiddle.

Dear friends, entirely different worlds reveal themselves. It is not only a difference in the sound of a flute and a string instrument; it is something totally different. And if you are a true composer, you of course can only express certain things by way of wind instruments, and other things by way of string instruments; and if you mix them up it goes against the spirit of music. Yet both belong together. You cannot imagine a modern orchestra – and when I say 'modern' I mean since the middle of the eighteenth century – you cannot imagine a modern orchestra without the wind and the string instruments. And you will then more and more learn to realise that the wind instruments are always starting, questioning, describing, whereas the string instruments are answering; they are pacifying, they are harmonising, they are forming out. In this question and answer, in this beginning and ending, in this interplay of these two instrument types, more or less all music can reveal itself. And not only accompanying it, but forming it, are the percussion instruments that beat the tact and rhythm. Again, we see how with this the totality of human existence is represented.

Let us return to the wind instrument and ask ourselves, what is it? How does such a simple pipe come into being? I don't mean how is it formed and made by a human being, but how does this form come into existence? How ever did the form of a horn arise, or the form of a trumpet? How was a flute or an oboe designed? These instruments, dear friends, belong to the human mouth. They are played with the help of the human mouth, be it the lips or the tongue or the whole of the mouth, and they are always played in such a way that it is as if the human voice would continue into the outer world. One can say that all wind instruments are nothing other than the continuation of this inner strength, the inner effort and the inner form that produces the human voice, be it sound or speech. But we see that what the heart and lungs and windpipe and larynx and mouth produce, together with the teeth and tongue and lips, this is, so to speak, formed and formulated anew. These are the wind instruments in all their various and differing forms. But why is it that these wind instruments, if they really come out of this rhythmical system, if they are a continuation of the rhythm of human existence and are formulated out of the human voice, why are they connected with melody and melos?

There are two kinds of wind instruments: the woodwinds and the brass winds. You can define the woodwinds as those that are more related to human feeling, to human emotions. Imagine a shepherd walking over the fields, playing the pipe; or imagine someone sitting, brooding about their life and existence, and expressing this by playing a primitive mouth organ: this is the task of the woodwinds. It is different with the brass winds: you would not think of someone quietly contemplating their feelings while blowing a trumpet. The brass winds come more from the lower parts of the human being, where the will forces have their seat, and where they drive human feelings outwards. Yet all the woodwinds are instruments of melody: you cannot play anything else on them but a follow-up – one note after the other. All this together becomes a melos, and this is a trend of thought.

Dear friends, this is one of the secrets of the wind instruments: that they display, in a form of nakedness as it were, the meaning and sense of willing and feeling. The melos rises up like a form that was clothed, and then reveals what before was hidden. The wind instruments are instruments of revelation for the hidden thoughts that lie in our feeling and willing, they perform something that rises from below upwards. In Greek times wind instruments were used to play the music of Dionysos. The Greek aulos for instance was played to bring about the wild dances in the Orphic mysteries.[3] Human beings were made ecstatic by the sounds of the aulos. They left their bodies and sheaths behind, rising up with the melos.

You will never see Apollo play the aulos. Apollo and

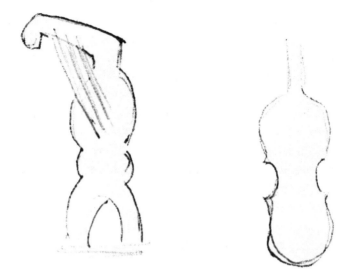

his son, Orpheus, are either playing the lyre or another string instrument. If you look at the pictures painted on ancient Greek vases, you will always find Apollo as the lord of the string instruments, the lyre or the gitara. You will find similar string instruments in ancient Egypt, and even further back in Sumeria. What does this mean? It is very strange. Some of these instruments have the following form: you find here a human head, a neck, a chest and two legs, with the strings extending downwards from the neck to the chest, as though alluding to the fact that the string instruments have come about out of the human being.

But the question is, how?

It is obvious that the very peculiar form of a violin, to take just one example, is not something that humanity thought out, although it is something that human beings think. You find a shape exactly like this on the island of Delos, in the most primitive human-made sculptures dating back to the third and fourth millennium before

Christ. I have the impression, dear friends, that what I have said to you about Dionysos and the wind instruments has to be developed in the following way: the human being expresses themselves by way of the wind instruments, the soul is reaching out, and this is 'the question'.

By way of a brief detour, there is a wonderful lecture that Rudolf Steiner gave in 1923 in which he describes what the meaning of birdsong actually is.[4] He explains that especially in the spring and summer, when the song of the birds is increasing, it reaches up in its melody into the far widths of the world, and from there it resounds (you can also say it is reflected) and brings to the earth spiritual forms from the cosmos. One has to imagine that the birds sing and their voices are carried out into the widths of the world where they take on the formative powers from the cosmos and bring them down to earth. Out of these formative powers, the Gestalt, the outer forms of all the animals, are brought about.

Something similar holds good for the interplay between the string and the wind instrument. If we have here the simplest possible wind instrument, it is the air within the sheath of wood or metal that gives rise to the sound. A string instrument, however, is different. A string instrument has a sound box, but it is not the air within the box that is responsible for the sound, it is the vibrating string. How does a wind instrument therefore transform into a string instrument? You can imagine it, dear friends, as a process of metamorphosis similar to the metamorphosis of long bones into the bones of the skulls as Rudolf Steiner has described it. If you open up and enlarge the sheath of the wind instrument, you will see that it becomes the sound box of the string instrument; and the air within hardens as it were and becomes the string. With this what was inside (the air) has become outside (the string), and what was outside has become inside in the sound box of a string

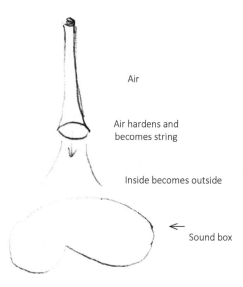

Air

Air hardens and
becomes string

Inside becomes outside

← Sound box

instrument. The string instrument is the answer to the
question posed by the wind instrument. The answer to the
question of Dionysos is Apollo.

And now read what Rudolf Steiner has to say about
the birth of the string instrument in the third lecture of
Christ and the Spiritual World. He has already described the
three pre-earthly deeds of the Christ – the harmonising of
thinking, feeling and willing – performed by the being who
in ancient Greece was considered to be Apollo. He goes
on to say how it is Apollo who brings about the harmony
of thinking, feeling and willing and how in the third pre-
earthly deed of Christ lies the source for all that gradually
developed as string instruments.[5] It has nothing to do with
the wind instruments because the wind instruments are of
an entirely different type; they do not harmonise, whereas
the string instruments they are the great harmonisers.
Following this, Steiner points to King Midas who was born
with huge ears because he was unable, in his pre-earthly

existence, to hear the string music of Apollo. But what does this mean, dear friends? When we sing, when we express our willing and feeling by means of wind instruments, this also rises up like the song of the birds rises up into the cosmos: the sound of the wind instruments rises up to the dome of our skull and from the dome of our skull it resounds. It resounds into 'Gestalt', into bodily form; it resounds according to principles I have indicated here. Then you find that all the string instruments, however different they may be, that every string instrument is in fact nothing else but a metamorphosis or a variation of our nervous system.

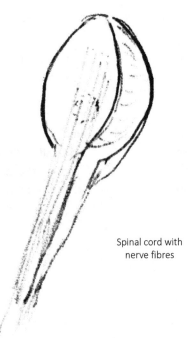

Brain

Spinal cord with
nerve fibres

Sketch of a string instrument

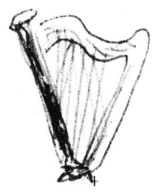

Sketch of a harp

Take a string instrument and consider its form. It is indeed an image of the brain, with the spine and the spinal cord cut in half and a few strings, a few nerve fibres, fixed to it. If you take a harp, for example, you find in this nothing other than the typical form that is to be found in certain parts of the brain and the nervous system.

Without going into details, we have a body of resonance that, like the song of the birds, brings down formative powers from the cosmos; the wind instruments, rising up, bring down the formative powers of the skull and brain that come out of the cosmos, and then all the different string instruments come about. This is Apollo.

Remember that the son of Apollo is Orpheus. Rudolf Steiner speaks about Orpheus in 1909[6] and 1913[7] in a very special way. He describes Orpheus as one of the bodhisattvas who during the third Post-Atlantean period was, so to speak, the king of the bards in Northern Europe. He instructed humanity in this part of the earth in music to prepare in their sentient soul the coming of logical thinking. This Apollo-Orpheus then incarnated again, but now in a much deeper, much more human way, as the Greek Orpheus. Again he is playing a string instrument.

Rudolf Steiner says of him that he is the founder of all the Greek mysteries; each one of the Greek mysteries goes back to Orpheus.

I cannot now go into the mythology of Orpheus and Eurydice, for it might take us much too far back. But I would only like to indicate, dear friends, how the whole of Greek civilisation was permeated by the element of music, by the interplay of Dionysos and Apollo as brought about by the works and deeds of Orpheus. If we now come forward a few steps in history, we find that Greek music disappears. The last music that was still formed by cosmic music, by the music of the spheres, disappears as the Word of Worlds enters earthly ground. As the sun shone through this earth, the stars of music faded away. Then, between the third and fifth centuries after Christ, the first three simple steps are made in Europe to recall the musical element. Gregorian song gradually developed and music started to take hold of humanity once more. Then, suddenly, in the tenth and eleventh centuries, musical script again developed. If some of you were to study how, out of Gregorian song a new type of music came about, you might consider that something significant must have happened, because it could not have come about simply out of itself.

To grasp what came about we need to pay attention to the signs of history in the way that Rudolf Steiner suggested: we should try to understand history as symptomatology, as a result of hidden or underlying processes. When you really study what happened around people like Bernhard of Clairvaux in connection with music, what happened for instance in the school of St Gallen in the tenth and eleventh centuries, and from the results of what the Irish and Scottish monks brought into Europe, you might ask, perhaps another Orpheus has appeared who has made this possible? Then your inner eye could look to a figure like Lohengrin, and see how, in the tenth century, he came out of the Castle of the Grail as a metamorphosis of what had been alive before in Orpheus. Lohengrin does not enter the underworld as Orpheus did, but like Apollo he comes from the north to the south to help another Eurydice. He is the new incarnation of what evolves as the music of the high and late Middle Ages, and which later finds its culmination at one special point: the music of Johann Sebastian Bach. When all of this draws together, then we see modern music unfolding from this point onwards. We are actually still in this process, a process that will still have to develop and unfold.

That Lohengrin is connected with the swan, dear friends, is not only due to the fact that a spiritual being, his Eurydice, is accompanying him. It is also because the swan in its form is the archetypal image of the string instrument. You can almost see how its body is hidden in it. This bird is nothing less than the form of our brain, and the form of the cosmos. From these indications one can understand how the song of the birds is rising up and returning, and how out of this all the string instruments are born. And one can begin to understand how this harmonising element rises up as a new Orphic stream within Europe out of the Castle of the Grail.

And what is behind all this?

When Rudolf Steiner, in the lecture that I have referred to above, describes Apollo before actually naming him, he speaks about a being who in his powerful form of light can overcome the might of the dragon. So that behind Apollo, behind Orpheus, behind Lohengrin, there stands the archangelic being of Michael, and through him the one who permeates and harmonises the human forces of thinking, feeling and willing: the being of the Nathan Jesus.

At the beginning of European civilisation, during the fourth century after Christ, the cosmic intelligence gradually descended to Earth. Until then it had been ruled by Michael, but then it fell away from him and incorporated itself into humanity, it became human intelligence. But this was not the only development, because if this cosmic intelligence can be permeated by what we call the Holy Spirit, then it is not human intelligence, it is music. And the rise of music, dear friends, during the last two centuries is the human answer to the form of cosmic intelligence, because music is the expression of the Holy Spirit. It is not merely symbolic that in pictures of the Middle Ages the angels are singing and playing instruments. This is the truth. The whole of the angelic world sounds forth with music, and this sounding forth of the choir of the angels presents to us the wonder and the miracles of the Holy Spirit.

This is what we can gradually learn to understand when we live within the substance of Whitsun. It is the music of the angelic world, and through this music the power, the might and the forces of healing of the Holy Spirit reveal themselves. And now you will understand why I wanted to try, on Whit Sunday, to lead you along this path of thought.

Music in
Curative Education

Notes from a lecture, Glencraig, July 6, 1958

We are treading almost completely new ground when we speak of music therapy. I wrote an article for the book *Musik in der Medizin* [Music in Medicine],[1] but what is known today about music therapy in America, Sweden and Great Britain, is to my mind a poor show of this very important therapeutic field.

Rudolf Steiner spoke about music in a very special way. In his two lectures he states that music is not of the physical world, that you cannot in fact hear music.[2] You can experience sound or noise or tone. In his course on tone eurythmy Rudolf Steiner also states that you cannot hear music, rather music is what you experience between two tones.[3]

So what do we hear? The world of hearing can be expressed in the following levels:

Noise
Sound [*Klang*]
Speech sound [*Laut*]
Tone

Speech sound is made by any living or ensouled being,

while tone can only be produced by the singing human voice or a musical instrument.

Let us look at each element by itself.

We need a constant and reassuring noise as a foundation for our existence. With it we know we are not alone. One could state that the sense of touch and the sense of noise are two related experiences. Noise can touch us so severely, that it can literally shake and shatter bones. Noise can destroy our physical existence.

Where the chaos of noise becomes more structured, like a crystal compared to an ordinary stone, there noise turns into sound. Indeed, in everything that lives sound is working, everything that has an etheric body is built by sound. All that today's physics knows about the realm of hearing has to do with this. Pythagoras wrote about it, Hans Kayser[4] writes about it today.

In speech sound the soul wants to express itself. It wants to convey its surprise, its wonder, its desire, its feelings – the sounds A or E or S and T or B express meaning.

Tone expresses in the realm of hearing what in mathematics can be expressed by the number one, the number in whom all other members are contained. Within tone all other elements are contained. Tone is universal, yet it is only very rarely experienced in its true nature as real tone. In experiencing tone I experience something like the 'I AM' of the other person. According to Rudolf Steiner, tone opens up and in each single tone the melos reveals itself.

Let us summarise these four elements:

Noise	sense of touch
Sound	sense of life
Speech sound	sense of movement
Tone	sense of equilibrium

How do we hear noise? As well as with the ear, drum and ossicles, we hear noise with the whole of our skin. It is a sense organ that extends all over the body.

How do we hear sound? There is the inner ear with its semi-circular canals and the organ of Corti. There is the cerebrospinal fluid, which resounds rhythmically in the rhythm of breath and pulse beat, the rhythm of one to four (72 to 18 per minute).

With the help of our larynx alone we are able to perceive speech sound coming from a living being. The larynx, in connection with our inner ear, is the organ that enables us to understand what the sound of ensouled beings wants to express.

The perception of tone has to do with the so-called motor-nerves system. In the lecture he gave on March 7, 1923, Rudolf Steiner states that we cannot in fact hear tone, rather we hear the music in between the tones.[5]

I would now like to add a few words about musical instruments. There are three types: wind instruments, string instruments and percussion instruments, of which the first two are the main types. From early on in our evolution instruments have accompanied humanity. It was the elemental beings, working through human hands, who created them. The wind instruments were there first, the string instruments came much later. Through wind instruments, humanity tried to express what was only in itself: the breath that can be played by the fingers. Later came the string instruments. What resounds in the human skull was reflected and became the various forms of the string instruments. The body of the lute, for instance, still resembles this origin, the brain.

Listen to the song of the birds, there you have an example of how music was first and later form appears. You might say that all forms of the animals come from this. A tremendous world breath is expressed in music:

Out goes the major,
Back sounds the minor;
Out goes the melos,
Back sounds the harmony.

What came from Dionysos as the wind instruments sounded from the south and was answered from the north by Apollo (Michael) with the string instruments. The great question and answer, like the melos and harmony.

If you study the history of music in the tenth, eleventh and twelfth centuries, you find a new stream emerging from which we still draw today. This stream comes from Lohengrin, the new Orpheus, from the north. Throughout the ages music has been used as the expression of the Holy Spirit, changing its expressions according to the epochs and development of humanity. Thus, also, was Lohengrin sent in the dawn of a new era in which we still find ourselves today.

On Seeing and Hearing

Notes from a lecture, Vienna (presumably), July 17, 1927

Rudolf Steiner taught us not to look upon the various sensory processes from a fixed standpoint, as happens in science, but to go deeply into each single one and realise that they are separate from each other, that they are different worlds. He taught that we do not only perceive with the sense organs, but that the whole of the human being always takes part in the sensory process in one way or another. With this in mind we will here attempt in an aphoristic way to say something about seeing and hearing.

Let us observe a plant as it appears before us in the summer. Its flower has opened to the sun, its roots are buried deep in the earth and given over to all its processes. It is part of the earth realm. Yet none of this inner activity is visible to our eyes. We see a form before us that changes over time, but we can see that it has been shaped from without.

If we now look at the human body and try to find something within it that corresponds to the plant in blossom, then our attention is drawn to the eyes: our eyes appear as metamorphosed blossoms.

Just as the flower is ringed by sepals that start from the stem and then unfold in colourful petals with the ovaries and the filaments in their midst, so the eyes are the result of a comparable transformation. The optic nerves, unfolding as an inner skin for the eyes, could be compared to the sepals, and the retina, surrounded by the skin of blood-vessels on the outside, resemble the petals. The outer skin, the quickly hardening sclera, is like the transformed ovary.

If we now have a look at the path of metamorphosis taken by the root, it leads us to the so-called motor nerves, meaning all nerves that go to the muscles in our extremities. Just as the nerves spread around in the human body in fine divisions, so also do the roots permeate the earthly realm in order to perceive its processes.

Rudolf Steiner taught us that our auditory perceptions come about from these nerves, which are open to the surrounding world of tone. We can understand this better if we clarify for ourselves the processes of hearing and seeing. If we listen intently, be it to music, birdsong or the wind, we relax our muscles. We close our eyes, and our arms and legs relax. Our body then resembles a harp, which is open to the surrounding world of sound. But if we want to have a good look at the flight of a bird or at a distant mountain to observe details, we tense our muscles and open our eyes wide. We are relaxed in hearing and rigid in seeing.

If we look at how the eye and the ear came about in the evolution of the human body, we see that the eye has been pushed outwards from the structure of the brain. It grows forwards towards the skin while breaking through all the tissues, reshaping itself in such a way that it lets the light through unrestrained. The ear, however, which has been formed like a dimple within the skin of the head, strangulates itself here and travels into the inward side of the head, where it then continues to transform itself still surrounded by bones, so that it has completely withdrawn from the outer world.

Just as the eye, growing towards the outside world, is an organ for perception, the ear, which has withdrawn from the surrounding world, is an organ of memory.

The tones from the surrounding world are not perceived by the ear, but, as we have already described earlier, by the so-called motor-nerves. (From this point of view one can also understand the close contact between the cochlea and the labyrinth in the ear, the organs for hearing and balance.) Yet the process does not end in perception only; we must *understand* what we perceive. And just as we perceive tones within the element of our will, in the metabolism and limb system of our body, we understand them also in our body's domain of feeling, in the rhythmical system. The memory of what we have perceived through sounds, however, lies within the domain of thinking, in the sensory-nervous system. The cochlea is the organ of memory for all that is heard.

The process of seeing takes a different course. The eye is here the organ of perception. The understanding of what is seen only wakes up in us in the rhythmical part of our body, the memory of it in the metabolic-limb-system. So, the processes of seeing and hearing are polar opposites.

We can distinguish yet another metamorphosis of the eyes and ears if we observe the human organism.

If we carefully study the appendages of the ears in the way they are arranged, how the Eustachian tubes next to the middle ear descend into the throat and how the throat merges into the larynx like a cavern that becomes narrower downwards, then we would see that something similar happens in the female organism. The fallopian tubes descend in a similar fashion into the uterus, which in turn merges into the vagina while being rejuvenated as it goes down. The ovarian system, however, is the opposite image of the ear. One only needs to picture a primitive auditory vesicle of a lower vertebrate with its crista[1] and the otolith[2] and one will see the great similarity to an ovarian [Graafian] follicle.[3] If, on the other hand, we observe the eye, and see how both of its lachrymal canals[4] merge into the lachrymal sac and from the nasal tear duct into the nasal cavity, then we find as counter-image in the male organism the testicles, from which the seminal duct leads into the widened part of the male urethra which is surrounded by the penis. In the same way as the latter has three erectile tissues, so also has the nose three corresponding conchae or shells (one of which even has an 'erectile' tissue). How close the metamorphic connections are between the aforementioned structures may also be seen in a rare malformation sometimes occurring in relation to the eyes of human embryos. If both eyes have grown together (so-called cyclopia) a similar snout-like malformation resembling the nose (proboscis) will develop above both eyes. The image is clear: during the development, the testicles rise out of the cavity of the abdomen into the scrotum; they unite in the same way as both eyes grow into one: the penis is the counter image of the 'proboscis'. From this metamorphosis we can recognise the polar manner in which the organs belonging to both sensory processes are formed. The eye resembles the set of forms that are typically male, and the ear those which are typically female. What occurs separately according to the sexes in the lower part of the human being is united in the head.

If we now attempt to go more deeply into the correspondences presented here, we arrive at the fertilisation process. By uniting what is produced by the testicles and the ovary the foundation of the human body comes about. And we must ask another question: is there anything that could be seen to be the fruit of the processes of seeing and hearing? Rudolf Steiner explained that speech is an organism brought about by human beings that has essentially been formed out of tones, and these are based on the manifestation of the human astral body. Yet within each speech sound there is a hidden colour that lends it the right sound character. What surrounds the colours, on the other hand, is permeated by tones, and these can become perceptible to someone with attentive consciousness.

In this way a common world arises out of separate sexual organs: the human body. Yet from the unification of the sensory organs two worlds arise and become manifest: the world of tone and the world of colour. What has been separated according to the sexes by the human microcosm corresponds to the separation of the two macrocosmic worlds. Both find their origin in the event of the Fall, but from the time when the Logos united with the world around in the Mystery of Golgotha, the possibility for the unification of the separate human sexes has also been given.

The Four Stages of Hearing

Previously unpublished article written by Karl König in 1963

> For one who listens in stillness
> A soft sustaining tone
> Resounds through all the tones
> In the colourful earthly dream
> *Friedrich Schlegel*

The sound

In our previous considerations we continued to research the close relationship that exists between all that sounds and moves.[1] We discovered that muscles are activated by the *movement itself* and not by the hypothetical action of a motor nerve. 'Movement intentions', which we attempted to describe more precisely, showed themselves to be the actual 'movers'. They proved to be tonal formations.

In this way a bridge was built that attempted to connect two spheres that had hitherto been separate: that of movement and tonality. We began by building the bridge from the realm of movement. Now we must change over into the realm of tonality and begin building the bridge also from that side.

We found musical laws underpinning each movement, and were able to recognise a sound element at the core of all motor activity. How can the world of sound itself be structured? Is it possible to bring order into it through which it will show its movement character? Is motor activity hidden within the experience of hearing in the same way as that which resounds is included within each movement? These are questions which now will have to be scrutinised. Before we do this, however, we will have to occupy ourselves with the totality of what can be heard and what resounds.

The world of sound is mighty and all-encompassing. It extends beyond the boundaries of what we can hear as human beings, the lower frequencies passing over into infra-sound and the higher ones into ultra-sound. In between lies audible sound – what we can hear.

It is not justified to think that these three kinds of sound are distinguished by the limitations of our organ of hearing and that this division is in any way arbitrary. We are able to hear audible sound not because our ears are sensitive only to a specific range of frequencies, but because only the middle frequencies (between 16 and 10,000 Hertz) resound.[2]

Infrasound is experienced as vibration and a similar sensation is transmitted by ultrasound. The former arises in the inner regions of the earth, through earthquakes and the beat of the surf. There is always some trembling in the solid and fluid elements that brings about the manifestations of infrasound. Hubert Rohracher's thorough investigations have shown that the surface of the earth constantly makes a rhythmical micro-movement of about ten vibrations per second. The human body has the same frequency of micro-vibrations, so that the earth and human beings appear to be vibrating in a kind of unison.[3]

Audible sound, what human beings can hear, emerges out of this sea of vibrations. The deep tones of a double bass still have a vibrational quality that we can feel. As the frequency increases, the tone becomes sharper and clearer as it approaches the boundaries of ultrasound. Then it turns into a shrill, almost unbearable noise, like the wail of sirens.

These high frequencies, which can only be brought about artificially by electro-magnetic devices, can have destructive effects. When subjected to ultrasound animals and plants soon die: their organic structure is destroyed, it loses its shape and form. Here we refer to cosmic frequencies that are no longer bearable to organic life.

Sound and speech sounds, however, exist together in the middle region between infrasound and ultrasound. Sound becomes the basis of tone in which mathematical and geometrical harmonies appear. The whole cosmos resounds. Our physical body is surrounded and permeated by a continuous field of mechanical vibrations caused by solid, fluid and airy bodies. This sea of vibrations encloses our body, flowing around it and penetrating it. We experience the lower frequencies as vibrations, we hear the middle ones in speech sound and tone, and with ultrasound our soul trembles and our body is disturbed by the unbearably high frequencies.

This is the ocean of sound surrounding us like the air surrounds the sea.

Ferdinand Scheminsky[4] begins his thesis, *The World of Sound*, by saying:

> The word 'sound' can have two different meanings.
> Firstly, it is something subjective, which every individual can only experience for themselves, namely the sensation that is transmitted to the ear via the sense of hearing.

Scheminsky then distinguishes the subjective quality from one that he calls objective, namely the physical processes that underlie the sense of hearing. With this statement he makes the same erroneous division that is still being made in the fields of physiology and psychology. Why would a musical sound be less 'objective' than a mechanical vibration? The fact that we need a sense organ in order to perceive a tone does not mean that this tone originates from that sense organ. The water that flows from the well into my cup was not formed inside the cup, although I would not be able to catch it without it. Similarly, the tone appears to the ear but is present in exactly the same way without it.

Nevertheless, I can describe sound from two sides: on the one hand it is the field of all mechanical vibrations and their inherent laws, while on the other it is the endless range of musical sounds, speech sounds, tones and noises that could change into experiences of vibrations and heart-rending sensations. Yet all of this is a self-contained unit in which human beings and animals are embedded, and of which only a part can be experienced while the rest can only be surmised.

Splitting up this unified world artificially led to an untold disaster that can only be designated as the 'fall' of all knowledge: the division between subjective and objective in the realm of the senses.[5]

This disaster also brought about the division between movement and musical sound, between that which brings forth sound and that which perceives sound. It is this division that we try to overcome by building the bridge about which we spoke at the start of this section.

The ocean of sound is the archetypal sea from which all that moves and all that resounds arises. Sound that permeates the world is the same substance out of which movement patterns and sound pictures appear in the world.

The poet Gerhart Hauptmann once expressed this in this way:

You will soon hear tones in the noise of the eternal
    rushing of the sea!
The primal sea of the kingdom of air, wedded to the
    primal sea of water,
To the primal sea of the soul, both, in turn, wedded.
You hear symphonies by the mighty master of tones.
Such symphonies release the tongue to the universe,
Transforming all sorrowful existence into bliss.
And you surmise the power of a sense that is a tiny
    particle
Of the faculty that senses the universe into which
    everything flows:
It is the sense of hearing.
Unrecognized today in the vastness of the power of
    manifestations
It has the key power over the all- powerful holy worlds.
Hail to you, o seer, you see!
And no less Hail to you, o listener,
You who can hear in the night
How the surge of the eternal tides comes and goes.[6]

Distinctions in the realm of sound

The ocean of sound is like an undifferentiated matrix from which the auditory pictures arise. Scheminsky, in his thesis cited earlier, distinguishes three such pictures:

> Simple soundscapes lead to the experience of pure tone, the composite sound with a regular structure leads to the experience of sound, while composite vibrations with an irregular structure call up the impression of noise.

Yet he also admits that acoustics makes use of these designations:

The latter concepts are also used in physical acoustics, although, strictly speaking, one can only speak of a simple and a composite vibration in a physical sense, and of tone, sound and noise only in the sense of an experience of sound.

Therefore, the division into two elements is here not at all applicable either, and tone, sound and noise are simply phenomena that can be described physically and physiologically.

The usual subdivision of that which sounds as presented above is only partially correct. Scheminsky himself says that:

> The word 'tone' in the sense of a sensation can in fact have two different meanings. Physically, tone signifies a simple vibration. Musically, however, the tone of a violin, a flute, or any other instrument is really a musical sound, as it consists of a large number of overtones accompanying the basic tone. Physically these tones can only be designated as sounds and yet they are tones.

Here, confusion arises due to the unhelpful subdivision into subjective and objective. Tone is the element from which all that is musical is built up and will therefore resound. Every tone, therefore, is also sound, but it is more than that. It has overcome sound and is experienced as a unity when it is perceived. Tone is not a simple, but rather a complex, sound structure that is so complete that it was able to return to the whole.

Apart from noise, sound and tone, a further element within the realm of the audible should be distinguished: speech sound or 'voice'. We know the speech sounds of our language intimately, but we do not acknowledge their independence as manifestations of sound, which cannot be designated as either tones, sounds or noises. They appear in the form of consonants and vowels, and just like tones they have a very complex structure made up out of very diverse sounds.

Rudolf Steiner always distinguished between tone and speech sound, and for this reason spoke about two forms of eurythmy: speech or 'voice' eurythmy and tone eurythmy, the former being the expression of speech, the latter the representation of music.

Our attempt to distinguish the various elements of the audible has so far led to four quite distinct manifestations, namely: noise, sound, speech sound and tone. The wisdom of language gives us these four designations because its genius knows much better than we do what can be distinguished in the realm of the audible. The diagram below gives us an initial picture of the field of hearing to which we will now turn.

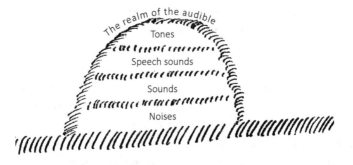

The ocean of sound

The realm of noise is the first to emerge out of the ocean of sound. It is the endless manifoldness that constantly surrounds and permeates us and offers those of us who can hear it a continuous assurance of our existence and presence in the here and now. The world is never silent for human beings who can hear. Even stillness can be heard because there is no end to noise. Noise is not the same as din. Noise is the rushing of the wind, the crackling of fire, the creaking of the stairs, the rattling of the window, the grinding of the wheels. It is the familiar footstep of the wife and the friend, the distant voices of the street, the beating of the heart, the whistling of the air and much, much more. It is the world that can be heard in the things and beings that surround us. Noise does not even leave alone the one who is lonely. Only a person who is deaf has to do without it and as a result they can sometimes become fearful and wary.

Noises are like waves that well up out of the ocean of sound. Usually they beat on the shores of our existence like a gentle surf, but sometimes they rise to a mighty height and their constant presence can become an unspeakable torture. The world of machines has penetrated the sphere of noise and has transformed it into an alarming relentlessness.

Noise can turn into sound. Sound manifests when the galloping of a horse resounds on the road in regular harmony, when the smith's hammer beats the metal rhythmically, or when the clapper of a bell hits the shell. Every noise that appears in regular repetition can either become sound or din. Undifferentiated and arhythmical noise remains chaotic to our ears. It becomes something different as soon as it begins to become ordered and regular. The rising and falling spray of a Roman fountain becomes sound. The rushing river becomes sound. The rhythmically beaten drum or tympanum, the drops that are steadily falling on the rock, all bring forth sound.

Sound pervades all living forms and structures. Hans Kayser describes the inner world of sound as the harmony that permeates all beings.[7] It has the power to give form. It works in the creation of plants as well as of animals and human beings. Its laws of harmony pervade works of architecture and sculpture. The path of the stars is regulated by the law of sound, and in the song of birds and human beings it is elevated to its most beautiful expression. Noise is outside and is all the time being manifested. Sound, however, works in secret. It forms and shapes, using mathematics and geometry as a secret harmonious force that permeates all that lives.

When sound becomes manifest in the resounding human voice and in the tone-filled utterings of animals, then it becomes speech sound. This transition has a significance similar to that of the transformation of noise into sound. The singing of birds and the bleating of lambs, the whinnying of horses, the barking of dogs, the roaring of lions are all speech sound structures. These are intensified in human beings in the formation of vowels and consonants, which form words and sentences in manifold combinations. Only human beings and animals can produce speech sounds.

Vowels have a stronger sound character, whereas consonants have clear elements of noise which determines them. The voiced consonants incline more towards the vowels and therefore also to sound; the voiceless consonants have a definite noise-character. All human speech as well as animal 'voices', however, are built up out of speech sound elements that can be distinguished in relation to sound as well as to tone.

Pure, true tone can only come forth from a human voice and permeate the listener with its radiating beauty provided it reaches its highest and most melodious level. When we speak about tone we have reached the realm of music; there are no other tones than those of music. This is why it has a special place among the arts. Music makes manifest much more clearly that the existence of nature and its creatures is complemented and enriched by the realm of art. Music is perfection in the realm of the audible and with it we have therefore reached the highest sphere of all that human beings can here.

Thus we meet a fourfold world of the audible and this division is by no means arbitrary: it has grown out of the world of what can be heard. Noise is an amorphous sound. It remains shapeless because it is not being carried by any rhythm. As soon as rhythmical sequences infiltrate noise, its amorphous shape changes into a crystalline form. In this form it is present in organic structures, it helps to shape them and begins to resound wherever life flows. Speech sounds arise wherever sensory and soul elements wish to be expressed. The sphere of voice and speech sounds ranges from the utterances of the animals to human speech and language.

Only the self can rise to tone. Beings with self-awareness, such as human beings, who become conscious of feelings and sensations and can reflect on them, begin to create musical tools. The feeling that reflects back to itself, the sensation that takes hold of itself and becomes aware of its sadness and joy, its foreboding and devotion, is the creator of musical instruments. Human beings coax tones out of this with the help of rhythmically moving lips and fingers, while pouring their own breath into it as the stream of substance. The pure, musical tone is something audible, surpassing speech sound because it brings order into sound in such a way that it becomes something new and consistent.

Summarising the above we now see:

1. Noise as an expression of amorphous structures.
2. Sound as an expression of organic forms.
3. Speech sound (voice) as an expression of the soul.
4. Tone as an expression of taking hold of oneself spiritually.

Described in this way, the audible appears as something that adapts itself to the layers of what is human and beyond. It is no longer an arbitrary thing, rather it is intrinsic part of the whole of nature.

The experience of hearing

If we now attempt to identify which sense organs belong to the four stages of the audible it will be impossible to link this to the current theories about hearing. The assumptions of these hypotheses are so fundamentally wrong that any questions and problems arising from them do not have any actual validity, only a semblance of it. I do not intend to go into these critical questions of knowledge here. Some philosophers, physiologists and neurologists have already begun to see these things in a new light, but it will be a long time before the indications of Rudolf Steiner[8] or Erwin Straus[9] for example are taken up.

It will not be possible to give the audible the place it deserves within existence if noise, sound, voice and tone are assigned a merely subjective character that is only present in perception but not in reality. The ear then becomes an instrument that conducts sound, with the mechanical sound waves transformed in such a way that they appear as auditory perceptions with the help of the hearing apparatus and a certain part of the brain. This assumption is causing such insurmountable difficulties for present day physiology in that it assigns to the ear the position of being the sole receptive organ for the endless fullness of what is audible.

The ear is not just an isolated sense organ and the only receptor for all that is audible. It is connected with other organic systems that need to be considered as part of a broader framework. It is therefore able to serve different functions.

The outer ear, for instance, is part of the skin and so belongs to the entire covering of the body. The outer auditory canal, which leads to the eardrum, and parts of the outer ear are made up of cartilaginous tissue, and the eardrum itself is inserted into a ring of bones. The auditory ossicles (three little bones called the hammer, the anvil and the stirrup) lie behind this in the middle-ear cavity. The organ of hearing is therefore connected with the entire support structure of our body, namely the skeleton and its many limbs.

Two muscles belong to the auditory ossicles, and while these muscles are very small and inconspicuous they nevertheless belong to the entire muscular system of the skeleton. The middle ear itself is a canal that forms an intimate connection with the throat, the mouth and the larynx via the Eustachian tube.

The inner ear with its complicated form, hence its name 'labyrinth', is embedded within the skull bone. Lymph-fluid travels through it and flows around it and thus it is part of the entire fluid organism of the human body. The labyrinth is also the sense organ connected to the auditory nerve, which, in turn, is part of the entire nervous system.

From this we can see that the ear is embedded within many other organic systems that extend into the ear and permeate it. The skin, the bones, the muscles, the nerves, the fluid system and the breathing and digestive systems are all closely connected with the ear.

It will only be possible to have a correct concept of how to perceive all that is audible if we follow up the many indications that Rudolf Steiner has given us about the function of the ears and the act of hearing. The following comment is, among others, fundamental to this:

> The ear really hurls the airborne tone back to the inner
> being of human beings in such a way that it separates out

> the air element; then, in that we hear it, the tone lives in the ether element. It is the ear's task ... to overcome the tone's resounding in the air and to hurl the pure etheric experience of tone back into our inner being. The ear is a reflecting instrument for the sensation of tone.[10]

The ear should therefore not be seen as an organ that simply transforms air into sound, but rather a structure that frees the tone from its covering of air and allows it to be lifted out of it. The ear reflects this liberated tone. In the realm of the audible, however, reflection is resonance. The ear is an organ for resonance, and the main purpose of the so-called 'sound-conducting' organs, such as the outer ear, the eardrum and the auditory ossicles, is to prevent the air from getting into the middle and inner ear. The vibrations are not guided but warded off. Under no circumstances should they reach the inner ear, because if they did they would be robbed of tone, voice and sound. Only when all vibrations come to an end, do voice and tone become audible.

Noise is in a position of transition. It is still so closely linked to sound that it cannot rise to pure auditory experience. It is easily mixed up with other sensory experiences, such as vibration. If I hold a tuning fork in my hand, it is hard to point out where the experience of vibration finishes and sound begins. This separation becomes even more complicated when I hold a buzzing insect in the hollow of my hand: now touch, buzzing, sounding and quivering all meld into one single sensory experience.

Why are sensations of sound, which are so closely linked with vibrations and experiences of touch, perceived in the inner ear? When we listen to low tones, do we not feel the vibrations coming in through our skin? And what about the shivering feeling we experience when an organ resounds with full registers? The whole body is then completely permeated by sound and tone, and we can have an immediate experience that we have become a sense organ from head to foot.

Such observations cannot be pushed aside because they point to actual experiences. The psychologists David Katz and Géza Révész extensively researched this question,[11] which led them to assume that there is an 'organ of vibration':

> The organ of vibration, which, in fact, is spread out
> over the whole body, as is also the case with the organ
> of touch, reacts to any stimulus of tone and noise. Being
> attentive, people with deaf-muteness are able to perceive
> the rhythm and volume of musical tones and even to
> distinguish their actual pitch more or less accurately.
> Apparently, the lower the tone, the lower down in the
> body the vibrations are experienced. Tones of the double
> bass, cello, bassoon, French horn etc. are perceived in
> the chest area, while the tones of the violin, flute, etc. are
> localised in the head.[12]

These indications make it even clearer that the whole body can be permeated by sound. Révész is even of the opinion that such experiences do not have any relationship to the impression being transmitted acoustically. The tones are not being heard, but their effect is being sensed and the sound belonging to it is experienced. Révész suggests that a wide field of research into musical experiences is available here.

> When it is said that music is 'gripping' or 'shattering' or
> forces you to move rhythmically, all this has to be taken
> much more literally than has previously been believed.
> Here we meet the immediate effect of strong vibrations
> on the vasomotor system in the body, which in those

of us who can hear determines our moods to a certain degree and in those who have deaf-muteness forms the pre-condition and, in fact, the totality of their musical experience.[13]

Here we come across the view that certain elements belonging to the experience of hearing affect the whole of the human body. The totality of the bodily organisation can become an instrument for resonance. It resonates, vibrates and is shaken by the elements that carry tones. This clarifies even more what was said earlier, namely that the ear is not an isolated organ but is incorporated into the various areas of our body and is connected to systems of resonance that differ from one another. Only once this is understood is it possible to describe the manifoldness of the experience of hearing as a functional achievement.

The four organs of hearing

The first stage is the perception of noise. This comes about whenever two objects or beings touch each other physically. We are not able to list all forms of noise because there are countless possibilities; it would take us too far just to name the most familiar ones. We all know them and have learnt to deal with them and to accept them as a daily accompaniment to our existence.

Would it really be possible that these endlessly diverse auditory impressions are only perceived in the ear? When I rub my hands, for instance, and follow up the subtle experience of what I can hear when doing this, I do not experience it in my ear at all. I will hear it there where it comes from. In fact, is it at all imaginable that this fine rubbing brings about such sound waves that they can make my eardrum and its organs vibrate? Physiologically this is not really acceptable. With what do we then hear this noise? Whence does the hearing sensation come of the crackling fire in the hearth, the blowing wind, the slamming door? Is it not embarrassing to think that I would assign all of this to the place where it originates although it is actually not there at all?

If you follow up noises with an open mind and observe their impact attentively you will soon notice that the area with the greatest sensitivity to noise lies within the outer ear. This structure is like the centre of a spiral that spreads out over the entire surface of the body like the main threads of a cobweb. The outer ear, as an organ of the skin and together with it, becomes the organ that senses noise. An understanding of this special structure will come about only when the close link between the outer ear and noise is recognised.

The outer auditory canal leads from the outer ear to the eardrum, and this is repeated in miniature within the body as a kind of web of noise spread out over the entire surface of the skin. The reason for this is that the eardrum is not the membrane of a tympanum, but a receptive organ for noise. There, at the eardrum, all noise breaks up and is prevented from going any further into the middle ear. In the event that the outer ear or the eardrum are lost, sound, speech sound and tone will be mixed up with noise, preventing clear hearing and causing all sounds to merge.

Certain kinds of fish and amphibians have an organ known as the lateral line. This is a series of circular areas that lie in a line behind each other; they can also spread out across the skull and along the lower and upper jaw. They look like primitive hearing organs and their nerves are of the same family as the hearing nerves. They serve to detect vibrations in the water and help fishes to orient themselves in currents and gain information about their environment. With some justification the lateral line can be thought of as serving the sense of 'touch from afar'. As the German zoologist Wolfgang von Buddenbrock writes:

> With their help solid bodies cannot only be perceived by the fish from some distance, they can also be correctly localised, so the fish can snap up marsupials, which can even be distinguished as to their size and the speed of their approach.[14]

The lateral line is a sense organ in the skin that is closely linked to the ear, and enables perception of current, pressure and noise. You can get an experience of this by surrendering yourself to the play of the waves on the beach, where noise, pressure, touch and rhythm flow together.

Scheminsky describes research by Knudsen[15] showing that sound can also be perceived by the sense of touch.

> The sensitivity of the organs of touch in the fingers, as is also the case with the ear, increases from the lower limit to the middle field of perceptible tremors that can be felt (250–500 Hertz), while decreasing again up to the higher limit ... The threshold of distinguishing the degree of the sensation of vibrations is practically as great as that of the sensation of sound.[16]

It thus becomes clear that the entire skin is a sense organ for sound, or in this case noise. And when Scheminsky adds 'Touch, however, is not hearing; the organs for touch lead to an experience of one's own quality', he is only partly right. So far it has not been conclusively proven that sound waves are felt via the sense of touch. It is the skin with its multitude of sensory 'bodies' that first receives them. Apart from this there is certainly a distinction between touch and hearing, but is it not a difference of degree? Is it not so that sound and voice gradually emerge out of a diffuse sensation of touch, impact and vibration that is very similar to noise?

The unfortunate theory of the specific sensory experiences still obstructs such a natural insight. Yet we begin to understand, step by step, that the whole human being hears and that the first step consists of the kind of perceptions of noise that are experienced over the entire skin and can flow together with perceptions of touch. The centre for this perception lies in the outer ear, the outer auditory canal and the eardrum.

If we now proceed to the experience of sound, we enter the sphere we called hidden. We should not mix up what we here mean by 'sound' with what is usually understood by 'sounds'. Here we are not speaking of a combination of several tones, for instance a triad, or a chord with five notes or a sixth, for these are harmonies or disharmonies. By 'sound' we mean the sphere of those formative forces that are active in all that lives and that carry within themselves the laws of harmony.

The experiences of vibrations researched by Katz and Révész and described earlier belong to the area of sound, as is also the case with the resounding of large or small bells, the tone of metal bars and plates, the low register of the organ, timpani, drums, and those sounds of the brass instruments that are no longer experienced as pure tones, but as vibrating sound masses. All that resounds and still has within itself an element of vibration is sound.

But when does it become our own experience? Here we should not look upon the ear as an isolated organ but try and understand the system of organs that vibrate with sound. The world of sound perception begins where the outer ear ends, behind the eardrum. The three small auditory bones, the hammer, the anvil and the stirrup, that stretch between the eardrum and the inner ear like an articulated bridge, form the resonance body for sound structures. Their vibrations are transferred to the so-called oval window, which then, in turn, causes the lymph fluid circulating in the labyrinth of the inner ear to vibrate.

The rhythmical movement of the fluid in the labyrinth caused by the auditory ossicles that are being moved by sound is one of the preconditions for the perception of sound. Additionally, the inner ear communicates indirectly with the inside of the skull through a special, sack-like protuberance known as the endolymphatic sac. The end of this small structure touches the lower side of the outer skin of the brain. This causes the cerebrospinal fluid, which is flowing up and down the spine and over the surface of the brain, to meet the fluid in the ear labyrinth.

The cerebrospinal fluid vibrates according to the rhythm of inhalation and exhalation and thus provides an accompanying beat to the varying movements of the fluid in the ear labyrinth. When breathing, human beings transfer the breathing rhythm to the fluid that is continually streaming and washing around in the brain and bone marrow within the skull and spine. The rhythm of the pulse that pervades the entire system of blood vessels is also included in this rhythm because the heart is situated rhythmically in the centre of the breathing as it moves up and down. The cerebrospinal fluid thus vibrates according to the rhythm of the breathing and pulse that permeates it. From the other side, however, comes the stream of fluid from the labyrinth of the inner ear that vibrates with the sensations of sound. Both rhythmical streams meet each other within the body because the sea of sound does not only permeate the ear, but also the whole of the breathing human being.

Let us take, for example, the thundering of a church organ. The sound penetrates us in a twofold way. It is drawn into the stream of the breath and from here it slightly changes the pulse of the blood. This is then communicated to the cerebrospinal fluid which vibrates to the rhythm of the sounds. This is the one stream. The other stream causes the auditory ossicles on the other side of the eardrum to vibrate rhythmically in the airspace of the middle ear and this vibration is then taken up by the lymph of the ear. The two streams meet where the ear fluid communicates with the fluid that flows around the brain.

The receptive organ for sound is thus formed by the pulse beat of the blood, the rhythm of the breathing, and the flow of cerebrospinal fluid, together with the vibration of the instrument of the middle and inner ear. Rhythm meets rhythm, and they are brought into tune with each other. They flow and surge and pulsate, bearing within them the laws of harmony of all living forms. Is it then so surprising that we are shaken when we hear the thundering of the organ or the sounding of trombones and the beat of the timpani? The whole of the human being is gripped and pervaded by it. We do not experience tone, but the creative power of the resounding tone formation.

Voice, or speech sound, arises from sound, and is the expression of the soul as it communicates something about itself. It originates in the larynx. Rudolf Steiner made a clear distinction between speech sound and tone when he spoke about the basic principles of the sense of the spoken word:

> A sound is a musical tone when, no matter how weakly, the overtones always sound with it. They are always perceived, even when they are practically inaudible. That is what accounts for the special quality of musical sound as contrasted with other kinds of sounds and noises. In melody, then, you have not only its single pitches but all the overtones as well ... Speech tones arise when a melody is instantaneously transformed into a harmony and then the fundamental tones are disregarded in favour

of the system of overtones. These overtones then convey the meaning of the tone 'A' or 'I'.[17]

The secret of a speech sound is the fact that a melody, built up of consecutive tones, is compressed and thus becomes a harmony of tones all sounding at the same time. The fundamentals, or keynotes, however, must be omitted from this so we can hear speech sounds. This is also how they originate.

The larynx is the organ that transforms melodies into harmonies. Together with the throat, tongue, teeth, gums, lips, oral and nasal cavities, the pharynx, the part of the throat that connects the nose and the mouth to the larynx, brings about the overtones whether we are here speaking about gum, lip, or tongue sounds. The larynx, on the other hand, holds back the keynotes, enabling the speech sound to be formed. The exhaled airstream is merely the matrix out of which the speech sound is formed. The false vocal cords (the outer folds protecting the true vocal cords) swallow up the keynotes.

It is only via the middle ear and the Eustachian tube connected to it that the ear is linked to the throat and thus also with the adjoining larynx. The middle ear continues over into the cavities at the back of the skull through the mastoid air cell system and thus becomes part of the whole of the skull. The larynx is itself a kind of skeleton, consisting of various cartilaginous structures. The outer ear is also permeated by cartilage formations, and the middle ear is surrounded by bones. The inner ear is embedded within the temporal bone and the auditory ossicles are part of the skeleton.

Thus, a very complicated structure of bones and cartilage comes about that sits on top of the larynx and carries the inner ear within itself as if inside a sensitive capsule. This work of architecture is not in any way an inflexible structure but is amazingly elastic, as is every bone. It has been known for a long time now that not only the air, but also bones conduct sound. Already in 1834, the German physician Ernst Heinrich Weber put a vibrating tuning fork on top of his head while at the same time closing his ears with a finger. He could clearly hear the tone of the tuning fork. Ever since that time the question of bone conduction has been discussed again and again and researched by many physiologists and oncologists. As a result, it has been proven that bone conduction is at least as important as air conduction in conveying sound.

Extremely high tones seem to be perceived exclusively via bone conduction. Certain parts of the skull vibrate at certain pitches. The Hungarian-American biophysicist Georg von Békésky did qualitative and quantitative research into the resonant qualities of the skull, according to which the skull has a resonance frequency of around 1,800 Hz. Below this frequency the whole of the head moves within a sea of the sound.[18] Various parts of the skull vibrate at different frequencies. In fact, the same author pointed out that bone conduction in the auditory ossicles gives up completely at frequencies above 2,000 Hz.

The consequence of this is that for most overtones only bone conduction is available and that only the combination of air and bone conduction can transmit complete musical impressions. Yet if air conduction is lacking, the fundamentals fall away and only the overtones, that is the speech sounds, can be heard. So here we find a third ear system that is built up out of the bony and cartilaginous support skeleton of the skull in such a way that it is in close connection with the larynx as it produces speech sounds.

It is for these reasons that we can hear our own voice so directly: once it is absorbed into the bone structure of the skull it is conducted to the ear. Yet it would be wrong to think that we hear speech sounds only with the inner ear.

The bones do not only conduct but also perceive speech sounds, in the same way as the skin perceives speech sounds and the rhythm of the cerebrospinal fluid perceives sound. Although the sounds that are hidden within a speech sound are perceived via the lymph in the ear labyrinth, the actual organ of perception for the speech sound is the spine that reaches down from the top of our shoulders and connects with the larynx, in as much as it consists of bone, cartilage, joints and connective tissue.

Tone is a completely new element. By this we mean that special region of the audible that is produced by human beings and is most likely fully accessible only to the human ear. This means that only human beings can hear tones not animals.

About the element of tone Rudolf Steiner says that there is a tone physiology only for sounds; there is none for tones. With the means customary today, one cannot grasp the element of music. If one does begin to speak about the musical element, it is thus necessary to avoid the ordinary concepts that otherwise use to grasp our world. He says:

> Musical experience does not actually exist in the same sense as sense experience does for the other senses.[19]

From these remarks is it clear that Rudolf Steiner equates tone with music; for him tone is a musical structure. This does not, however, mean that music only consists of tones. It carries all the different levels of the audible within itself, but tone only becomes visible in the realm of music. This is why it does not exist in the physical world as we know it. It only comes into being through the human voice or by instruments fashioned by human beings.

The special thing about music is that it recreates the highest member of its elements, tone, and adds it to speech sounds and to sound. This makes tone into something new that can hardly be grasped by the usual categories of knowledge at our disposal. In this way an area enters our customary world that already has a character of 'otherness'. The perception of tone is different from other sense perceptions such as of colour, smell, touch and noise, in that tone opens up a world that lies beyond the boundaries of the senses.

Yet there is hardly any doubt that tones are experienced within the innermost cells of the ear in the organ of Corti of the cochlea. I said 'experienced' and not 'perceived', because I am, initially, adhering to the indication by Rudolf Steiner that was quoted earlier where he says that the ear is a reflective organ for the experience of tone.

In the comparable anatomy of the ear, it is striking that only the highest animals, the mammals, have a fully developed cochlea. Even in songbirds the cochlea is only a short stalk, and in the rest of the vertebrates it is a small protuberance of the otherwise well-formed and fully developed labyrinth. This also shows that the possibility of experiencing tone is only granted to the highest stages of organic structures. Yet this does not mean that animals with a fully developed cochlea experience tone. We are only pointing out the parallels between tones developing out of speech sounds and sound, and the cochlea arising from the labyrinth.

Tone physiology is now able to prove beyond any doubt, through experiments and through tests of diseased ears, that different pitches are linked to particular places in the basilar membrane that lies within the cochlea. The lower tones, for example belong to the apex of the cochlea. It is possible to say with a degree of certainty that this 'belonging' is a form of resonance.

Apart from this classification, however, the physiology of the organ of Corti is still shrouded in mystery. Even Ranke is forced to confess:

The many correspondences between physics and perception, however, face serious limitations, for which the physics of the cochlea has as yet been unable to offer any understanding of what is actually perceived.[20]

This lack of ability is also connected with the attempt to place all perception of tone experiences within the organ of Corti. Physiological acoustics faces particularly insurmountable difficulties in the experience of harmony, of mixed sounds that pass over into each other and yet are experienced as if separate, and of instruments that sound simultaneously yet can clearly be distinguished from each other, because the lymph fluid moves much too slowly to be able to process this plethora of stimuli.

Where else, then, do we perceive tones? Rudolf Steiner gives an almost unambiguous answer to this, as we have already pointed out in the previous chapter. There he says:

The sense organisation in the ear is inwardly connected in a very delicate way with all the nerves which present-day physiology calls motor nerves, but which are in fact the same thing as sensory nerves; so that all we experience as audible is perceived by the nerve strands embedded in our limb organisation. Everything musical has to penetrate deep inside our organism first of all – and our ear nerves are organised for this – and in order to be perceived properly it has to seize hold of those nerves deep within our organism in which otherwise only the will is active.[21]

This indication directs us to the fourth organic system of all that is audible and which facilitates our experience of musical tones. The myriad of nerve fibres that take care of the organ of Corti connect with the auditory nerve (the *nervus acusticus*) and enter the brain. There they divide up anew, penetrating the various parts of the brain in the most diverse directions and linking up with the motor nerve fibres coming from other parts of the body. In this way a network of nerves comes about that is spread out over the whole of the body and that is not unlike an extremely complicated musical instrument. The nerves become the strings of a lyre that has its framework in the limbs and its bridge in the brain, to which both ears are connected via the auditory nerves.

This picture is at first only a hunch. It points to possibilities that will only be introduced into this area of research in the coming decades, but such ideas indicate the direction that our research should take. May the words of St Basil then again be heard and understood when he said:

> The body is a string instrument (a psaltery), made for
> the singing of hymns to our God. The actions of our
> body can become psalms, because it has been structured
> so harmoniously that even our movements become
> harmony.[22]

In this quotation what was revealed to us in our search for the organ of perception for musical tones is indicated from a different point of view. This will be able to guide the steps of our newly acquired knowledge into the next chapter.

Summarising, we can say that we have found four organic systems for the experience and perception of the fourfold world of what human beings can hear. We perceive the enormous variety of noises through our skin. The organ for these perceptions is formed by a network that is centered in the outer ear, the outer auditory canal and the eardrum, and is spread out over the entire surface of the body.

Sounds take hold of the auditory ossicles, as well as of the lymph fluid that flows into the ear labyrinth. Their rhythm passes over from here into the flow of the cerebrospinal fluid and in this way connects to the pulsing blood as well as to the breathing rhythm. Sound lives in the flow of the body fluids and in the coming and going of the breath.

A complicated structure lies over and above the larynx and its related organs which produce speech sounds: the entire cartilaginous and bony skeleton of the face and the head. Here it is especially the bone conduction that contributes to the perception of speech sounds. The ear and the larynx join via this supportive skeleton.

Lastly, we found that the perception of tone is achieved with the help of a network of nerves that is spread out over the entire body. They are connected to the inner ear via the auditory nerve (*nervus acusticus*) that goes into the brain, thus forming a string instrument with endless ramifications.

These four organic systems are also the archetypal forms of all musical instruments: from the 'sack' of the skin, via the wave-like rhythms of the air and the blood and the cerebrospinal fluid, and via the hollow form of the bony skull to the lyre of the outstretched nerves.

Thus, in as far as we begin to understand the bodily organisation in the right way, the human being becomes something that contains all musical instruments within its form: the human being is like a divine lyre. This saying by Claude de St Martin[23] is becoming ever more real:

> When, in your clearest moments, you have come so far
> that you hear the music of things, then all that is manifest
> will appear to you merely as a number of masks of the
> One.[24]

Yet the mask of the One becomes an instrument for the universe.

Music Therapy
in Curative Education

Article published in *Musik in der Medizin* [Music in Medicine] in 1958. It was later published in English in 1966 in *Aspects of Curative Education*.

Introduction

In 1846, Edouard Séguin, one of the originators of curative education, wrote in his work *The Moral, Hygienic and Educational Treatment of Idiots and Other Backward Children*:

> I have not yet seen any feeble-minded persons who did
> not show the greatest pleasure in listening to a piece
> of music. They react faster and more immediately to
> joyous and enlivening rhythms than to slow and sad
> ones. Some could be pacified when they were in a state
> of excitement by listening to a mournful song. On the
> other hand, lively and pronounced rhythms of drums
> and brasses cause movements in [those] who had
> never shown any before. On occasion I have even used
> military marches to enthuse or to encourage my pupils
> to spring, run or climb.[1]

These remarks – made more than one hundred years ago – clearly point to the general possibilities that music has and can have in curative education.

The Austrian psychologist Theodore Heller also writes in his manual:

> Under the influence of singing there awaken in the soul feelings of a higher nature which lift it above the mere material. Only singing imparts to festivities and celebrations the right mood of solemnity.[2]

There will hardly be a residential school or other educational institution for children in need of special care that will not use music as a means of pedagogy. Here, as elsewhere in life, music is a beneficial, enlivening and character-forming influence.

Séguin points mainly to the stimulating effects of music, Heller to its uplifting influence. One could still enumerate many other influences called forth by the power of music, such as the effects of tones on every human being, be they healthy or ill. Music can enthuse and invigorate, it can calm or create a mood of sadness. Music can imbue human beings with courage, but it can also paralyse them. We should not, however, regard all these possibilities as therapeutic effects. If we do this, we regard music as having nothing else but therapeutic powers.

There is yet little willingness to differentiate the way music therapy has been practised during the last three decades by American[3] and English[4] exponents. Music is used in a random fashion, and compositions from Schütz and Bach, Bartok and Schönberg tend to be regarded as the only kind of music. This brings about applications that are far removed from true music therapy. Thus, most of the papers published on the subject deal only with the general effects of music without even trying to touch upon specific questions of music therapy.

Composed music, be it orchestral, choral or chamber music, consists of so many different factors that analysis is hardly possible. Such differentiations as 'gay', 'sad', 'stimulating' or 'pacifying' are scientifically impermissible since they deal with too general an emotional sphere and are subject to much individual variation.

The first one to recognise this problem was Aleks Pontvik, who tried to find a new direction.[5] In the chapter 'From Psychoanalysis to Psychorhythmy'[6] he refers to the basic investigations of Hans Kayser, who for decades has been concerned in tracing the fundamentals of music and the nature of sound.[7]

With regard to formulating a new music therapy we must try first of all to analyse music into its archetypal elements and their effect on human beings. When these steps are accomplished, a general as well as a specific music therapy can be developed, for instance in the field of curative education. The former would endeavour to work in the direction of general effects, as indicated for example in the quotation of Séguin. A specific music therapy, however, would lay hold of specific forms of disability such as deafness, various forms of paralysis, psychotic and post-encephalitic conditions, and so on.

Only if we proceed systematically in this way can we hope to achieve useful and teachable results. We cannot start with the abundance of a symphony by Beethoven or Bruckner, but must begin instead with the single elements of music in order to study their effects on human beings.

This does not mean that the blessings of music should be withheld from sick people. It is only good and right that in hospitals and institutions concerts are given, that patients practise choir singing and even form a small orchestra. But these measures should as little be called music therapy as a good or a bad meal should be called a therapeutic measure. Just as every human being has to eat, so they can be given the blessing of music. A sick person, however, requires medicine, which is something different from food. In the same way, composed music is a kind of food for the soul, but music administered as medicine is basically different and requires an understanding of the archetypal elements of music.

The elements of music therapy

As long as we regard music as a purely aesthetic affair, we cannot achieve an understanding of its all-embracing greatness and effectiveness. Pontvik rightly referred to Kayser when he began systematising his forms of music therapy, because Kayser, following up on the indications of Baron von Thymus in the last century, had investigated the numerical laws of music and compared them with similar laws in the organic world. Kayser had succeeded, for example, in translating growth principles in the world of plants to certain basic harmonic values.[8]

Rudolf Steiner's hypothesis is even more comprehensive than Kayser's. He tries to understand music as a working principle that can be taken hold of in all spheres of life. Just as Kayser attempts to describe the morphological structure of music, so Steiner traces its physiology and psychology. He describes, for example, how in the course of human evolution the experience of music has changed. He especially refers to the experience of the intervals, to which he attributes a basic significance. He shows how in ancient times human beings had an experience of the seventh that, step by step, changed into the experience of the fifth, and then in more modern times into that of the third. Through this there arose a few hundred years ago the differentiation between the experience of major and minor, which is connected with the distinction between the major and minor third. Steiner points out that the child even today up to its ninth and tenth year lives entirely in the mood of the fifth and how this changes only after this age.[9]

Whoever has felt the soaring and weaving of music composed in the fifth and has then experienced the awakening element of the introduction of the fourth (for example, the Dutchman motive from Richard Wagner's opera) will try to follow up such indications.[10]

Steiner goes on to show that the experience of the major is closely connected with exhaling and that of the minor with inhaling.[11] This coincides with the indications of Goethe who regards major and minor as the polarities of music theory. Thus, for the soul, the experience of the major is a kind of exhaling, a widening out into the world. The experience of the minor, however, can be compared to the process of inhaling: the soul connects itself more intimately with the body. The extrovert can be described as the 'major' human being, the introvert as the 'minor' human being.

The above descriptions of musical elements are still of a rather general nature. When Goethe says that 'the audible in its broadest sense is infinite',[12] then we should take this very seriously, for he means thereby that sound – what is audible – works through the world in a way that is as comprehensive as light, for example: both are archetypal forces in nature and in humanity. Music therapy in the future will have to study the basic elements of what weaves through the world as sound until the working of melody, rhythm and harmony is understood. These are the three elements by which any musical phenomenon, if it is not a single tone, manifests itself as music.

Steiner has also made some fundamental observations in this area. He points out that not only is the ear receptive to sound, so too is the whole human being.[13] In our limbs we are susceptible and react directly to rhythm; in the sphere of breathing and circulation we experience harmony, and with our sensory-nervous system we comprehend melody.

The threefold human being, which Steiner describes from many points of view, thus becomes the expression of the three archetypal elements of what may be called World-music. When we realise that the power of willing belongs to the human limb-organisation, the element of feeling to the rhythmic organisation, and the element of thinking to the sensory-nervous system, the result is a first basis for the application of melody, harmony and rhythm in music.

That not only the organ of hearing but the whole human being is an instrument for the sensation of tone, becomes obvious from the otherwise incomprehensible findings of David Katz and Géza Révész regarding deaf people.[14] What these two authors postulate as vibration-sensation and vibration-organ are nothing other than the general music receptivity of the human organization, which is integrated into beat and rhythm through the limbs, harmony in the realm of the breath and melody through the ear.

Pontvik refers again and again to the findings of Katz and Révész to explain the effect of music on the unconscious. In reality it is only melody that we grasp with our full waking consciousness. It is therefore easiest for us to remember melodies and, by melody, to recall musical experience. Harmony requires active thinking in order to be grasped clearly, and rhythm is followed unconsciously in marching or dance, in the beating of time or some other motor activity.

Much detailed investigation will be required to verify these first indications, which have provided me with a well-proven working hypothesis based on decades of experience.

With this insight, it should now be obvious that true music therapy can only be exercised by music-making human beings and not by a record player, because only human beings are the instrument of the totality of music.

The record player, no matter how faithfully it reproduces sound, is not living music; it is, as it were, a memory of music: it can reawaken in the listener beautiful and elevated emotions, but it can never be a substitute for the direct effect of music as a therapeutic medium.

The record player has its justification in psychotherapy as a passive influence on the emotions. But when a much deeper influence is required, only music-making human beings – as singers, as instrument players, as performers of music in the field of movement – can work therapeutically. A singer works especially within the element of melody; when they play an instrument they work out of the sphere of harmony, and when they make music in the realm of movement, they rely especially on rhythm and beat. This characterises the three main forms of music therapy as:

1. Song
2. Instrumental music
3. Tone eurythmy

These three basic principles form the therapeutic medium whether used singly, combined in twos, or all together. It is perhaps easiest to show examples of the practical application of the above in the realm of curative education.

General music therapy in curative education

We have already pointed out that music should play an important part in the life of a curative-educational establishment, but that this should not be taken to mean music therapy in the proper sense of the word. Soothing sounds will calm the unrest of an excited child, whereas lively inspiring sounds will enliven a dreamy child. This fact does not belong to the realm of therapy but to simple life experience.

Yet even here we enter the border area between such life experience and therapeutic measures. In our schools and homes, for example, waking up children in the morning with music has become the rule. A cheerful melody played on the recorder or violin rouse the sleepers to face the day. In my experience such a musical sound upon waking avoids giving the children too strong a shock. For those children with epilepsy, it can even reduce the number and strength of seizures.

In the same way the evening concludes not only with the common evening song, but in each dormitory goodnight music is an important part of daily routine. For many children a bridge into sleep is built that normally they have difficulty in finding.

But a general music therapy only begins when the basic musical elements of melody, rhythm and harmony are directly applied to the individual child. A description of this was published some time ago by Julia Bort. She describes a music therapy where the three basic elements are used singly.[15]

Our own therapeutic research has shown, for example, that children suffering from a certain lack of concentration, who cannot keep their eyes still and who are so deeply involved in the experiences of smell and taste that they must sniff and lick everything, can be substantially helped by daily exercises in listening and singing simple tunes. The flight of thought, which in this case is the cause of the lack of concentration, is restrained through repeated listening to the course of the recurring melody. The melody brings order into the chaos of thought sequence. Such melody exercises can be practised either by singing or with woodwinds. Flutes, clarinets and recorders are those instruments that reproduce the melodic element at its purest.

If, however, a child is restless, not so much because of their disturbed thought-life but rather because of motor over-activity, so that they cannot keep their hands or feet still, but is constantly carried away by them, then rhythm will be the right musical agent. Just as Edouard Séguin already pointed to the influence of military marches, so in a refined and more subtle way musical rhythms can be applied. Whether to use the more soothing 3/4 beat or the enlivening 2/4 beat must be decided in individual cases. From the realm of speech one can introduce the will-inspiring iambus or the trochee working soothingly on the emotions to give aim and direction to the disturbed limb organisation. This makes it immediately understandable that percussion instruments such as drums, triangles and cymbals, are the true rhythm – and therefore will – instruments.

String instruments such as the violin, cello, harp and lyre bring the element of harmony to its purest expression. They work mainly in the rhythmic organisation of human beings, influencing breath and heartbeat and, through them, the emotional life. Children whose emotional life has been disturbed or even blocked through psycho-traumatic experiences in early childhood and who, because of this, live in a permanent state of anxiety are greatly helped by being bathed in sound consisting of sequences of pure harmonies. Chords played on two or more string instruments exercise a powerfully harmonising influence on a disturbed emotional life.

At this stage we must point to an instrument that, in the last three decades, has achieved a very special place in curative education, and which in fact has made possible certain techniques in music therapy. It is the lyre, built and proved by Lothar Gaertner and Edmund Pracht.[16] These lyres are string instruments of different sizes, ranging from one to several octaves. Because of the way they are built they have a particularly urgent, clear and carrying sound. I have often observed how children who refused to react to any other instrument would respond to the sound of the lyre.

As a stringed instrument, the sound of the lyre affects the emotions. The clarity of its tones, however, allows for the possibility of awakening true tone experiences where none were yet present. It has therefore been used with success in the treatment of deaf and hard-of-hearing children. Thus, the lyre is a valuable aid not only for general but also for special music therapy.

Special music therapy in curative education

Special music therapy refers to the application of music and its archetypal elements to particular medical conditions in the field of curative education. Special music therapy mostly involves group therapy and is directed towards the process of the disturbance itself, whereas general music therapy focuses on the individual person. Special music therapy tries to work out musical remedies for illness from a definite cause, whereas general music therapy selects from the all-embracing being of music those elements that can meet the disturbances of thinking or feeling in an individual child.

Music therapy and severe contact disturbances

In our schools during the last ten years we had the opportunity to observe a significant number of autistic, schizophrenic, pre-psychotic and post-encephalitic children. We succeeded in ordering the manifold symptoms in such a way that an underlying unity of these medical conditions can be assumed.[17] We could also show that there exist two main types, one showing mainly erethic and the other mainly torpid characteristics. The torpid type goes in the direction of what today is called juvenile schizophrenia, whereas conditions pertaining to encephalitis show predominantly erethic characteristics. We have, however, observed a series of cases where one condition can change into the other. This we take as proof of the underlying unity referred to above. Anatomically we regard the seat of the disturbance as being in the thalamus area. These conditions permitted us to show two further characteristic symptoms, which then gave us indications for a suitable music therapy. We found in erethic post-encephalitic children an intensified deep inhaling followed by forced exhaling, while in children with torpid schizophrenia the whole breathing process is shallow and reduced.

Since with schizophrenic children the disturbance relates mainly to sense-impressions, and with post-encephalitic children it is the motor area, we have tried to bring about a suitable music group therapy.[18]

With schizophrenic children where the emotional life is often as shallow as the breathing process, the following has been instituted. As quietly as possible, the children are led into a room illuminated by a weak red light. They are then encouraged to walk to the rhythm of simple music played on a lyre and a triangle. The beat becomes faster until the children begin to trot and run. Then the music is silenced, and the children are guided through eurythmic exercises of a strongly social character. Following this, intervals are played on the lyre, leading from the seventh to the fifth into the third. This concludes the group exercise. After this it was possible to observe a deepening of the breathing process and an enlivening of the children's emotions.

Group therapy for the erethic post-encephalitic children begins in a room filled with a dusky blue light. The children sit quietly and are encouraged to breathe in time to a simple drumbeat. The breathing then progresses to humming and then singing. This is followed by silence during which the children are shown a brightly illuminated picture, usually one of Raphael's Madonnas. After a time the picture is removed. The singing, humming and breathing exercises are then repeated in reverse order, and this concludes the group therapy.

With the first group we try to enliven the limb-motor sphere through breathing and the walking/running exercise; with the second group the breathing process is led into the region of sense experience through the use of the illuminated picture. Both therapies have proved particularly helpful with these two groups of children. Only the basic features of the therapy have been outlined here, and these can be altered in accordance with the age of the children and the means available.

Music therapy for paralysed children

Treatment and care of paralysed children has made significant steps forward during the last decade, particularly in the Western world. Physical therapy is often accompanied, supported and enlivened by music and singing,[19] and music often has a prominent place in the teaching of paralysed children in school.[20] Such measures, however, still belong to the area of musical life-experience.

When we tried to support the treatment of paralysed children by music therapy, we took our start from certain symptoms that are invariably found in connection with paralytic symptoms. There are typical emotional disturbances that accompany the various forms of paralysis: hemiplegic paralysis is often accompanied by hypomanic and depressive episodes; athetotic paralysis by uncontrollable outbursts; spastic paralysis by melancholic moods, and rigid paralysis by a phlegmatic apathy.

These connections between motor disability and emotional disturbance seemed to call for musical group therapy, which in our view was to be mainly a passive therapy. I have already reported extensively about this and shall give only the basic principles here.[21]

We try to bring the children into a state of complete relaxation that not only resolves the motor contractions but also those of the emotional sphere.

To this end we use a specially constructed oblong room with five windows, all of them on the short side; the other walls have no windows at all. Each window can be covered by differently coloured screens (blue, red, orange, yellow and green). About 8 feet (2½ metres) from the windows a white, translucent linen screen is stretched across the whole room in such a way that an object placed between the windows and the screen will throw multi-coloured shadows onto the screen.

During group therapy the children sit in rows facing the screen. Eurythmy is performed behind the screen creating a display of shadows in ever-changing form and colour. The performance is accompanied by a small orchestra that plays behind the audience. We usually use two or three lyres, a spinet and a small choir. Placing the orchestra behind the children allows the music to connect directly with their emotions. The music, specially composed for the purpose, is full of harmony since it is intended to work mainly on the rhythmic organism of the children.

The patients were given this sound- and colour-bath three or four times a week with highly satisfactory results: the children were noticeably relaxed following each treatment; cold hands and feet became pleasantly warm because of the improved blood circulation; emotions could be harmonised for days, and the group therapy relieved many of the paralysed children of their severe emotional disturbances.

Music therapy for deaf and near-deaf children

Acoustic methods in the education of deaf children have been known for a considerable time and tried again and again. The French physician Jean Marc Gaspard Itard wrote towards the end of the eighteenth century in his textbook on otology:

> Sound waves are the most decisive means of stimulating the ear and a re-enlivening of the sense of hearing cannot be achieved without their applications. All musical instruments which bring forth intensive tones can be used; the rich sound of bells as well as the beat of drums.[22]

Itard's suggestions have again and again been taken up, particularly by the Austrian medical doctor Viktor Urbantschitsch. But it is only recently that an active and dynamic education of deaf children has come to the fore, and the acoustic method is increasingly used.[23] In our residential schools this method of treatment was introduced many years ago. We discovered the basis for it in Steiner's comments on the nature of hearing. Years of experiments with deaf or near-deaf children showed that often the problem has less to do with the sense of hearing, than the possibility that listening has not been acquired or developed. We therefore begin every treatment with a step-by-step development of the faculty of listening.

To this end we mainly use the human voice and the lyre. In a quiet and slightly darkened room single tones are sung into the children's ears. This is a daily exercise, and after some time single intervals are played for the children on the lyre. Slowly the children learn to concentrate on this new world of sound and to experience things previously inaccessible. When a child has taken this step and learned to listen to the hitherto unknown sense-contents, much has been gained.

Slowly, high and low tones can be distinguished and intervals comprehended. One can then start the children on bringing forth tones and sequences of tones themselves. Gradually, the children acquire control of their breathing for speech and singing sounds. What is most important with these exercises is the continued application of human and instrumental voices, which alone keep awake the newly acquired faculty of listening.

We learned at the beginning to distinguish two groups of children. One are motor-excited and restless, disorganised in their activities and unable to control their limbs properly. These children are deaf for high and very high tones (high tone deafness), and their education in listening began with high-frequency tones. The lyre with its clear and penetrating sound was especially helpful here. Minor harmonies were mainly used to lead the children to an experience of their own bodily nature. The calming and harmonising of motor activities through active listening is most important with this group.

The second group of deaf children is characterised by languidness. Here we start with deep tones, progressively broadening the range of hearing upwards. Major harmonies are used for their activating and awakening effects. Activation of listening is required here, which then works back and enlivens the motor activity.[24]

Treatment of the whole human being is necessary because always the whole area of motor-activity is involved. As a result, there appears in this region either hypertrophic or hypotrophic characteristics, meaning that all action is either over- or under-developed, which disturbs the unfolding of the personality. Only when listening has been learned is a counter-pole created against over-activity or inactivity of the limb system. Only the world of sound can bring harmonisation here. When listening has been learned, rhythmic exercises with drums and percussion instruments lead to the co-ordination of restless limb movements.

Flute melodies on the other hand help apathetic children to concentrate and become conscious of the possibility of listening.

Needless to say, speech must play a most important part in the education of deaf people, but this is beyond the scope of this article. We are certain that acoustic treatments for deaf people are the best method.

All that has been said here can be only a sketch and an indication. The available space is much too limited to do justice to the ever-widening field of music therapy. It has been my task in this article not to describe the land that lies before us, but to point towards it. In conclusion, the following sketch may be a compass to those who, out of their own initiative, wish to enter the land of music therapy.

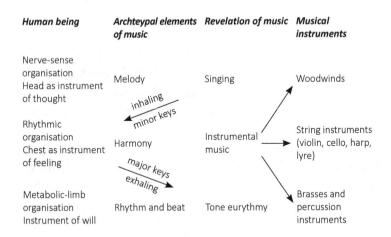

Human being	Archteypal elements of music	Revelation of music	Musical instruments
Nerve-sense organisation Head as instrument of thought	Melody	Singing	Woodwinds
	inhaling minor keys		
Rhythmic organisation Chest as instrument of feeling	Harmony	Instrumental music	String instruments (violin, cello, harp, lyre)
	major keys exhaling		
Metabolic-limb organisation Instrument of will	Rhythm and beat	Tone eurythmy	Brasses and percussion instruments

The Lyre

From *The Cresset*, Christmas, 1955

It is now almost thirty years ago that, through the collaboration of two men, one a musician and the other a sculptor, an entirely new musical instrument made its appearance in our civilisation. Although it is called a lyre, it is not the same as the Greek lyra. The Greek lyre was a string instrument made to accompany the rhapsodic declamations of priests and poets.[1] In many different forms it has been the companion of humanity throughout the ages: first as the Greek kithara and the Celtic chrotta, then in more recent times it changed into the harp, the virginal and the harpsichord. Even the modern piano is an intellectualised offspring of the old lyre.

The new lyre, however, has assumed a form that is much nearer to the archetypal idea from which all later forms of the lyre sprang. It has a simple wooden frame with a varying number of strings stretched across it. It is held against the chest, and the frame of the lyre can be seen as an extension of the architecture of the human chest where the twenty-four ribs enclose the rhythmical play of breath and pulse. When the strings are plucked to create the musical sound, it is the same phenomenon that occurs each time the human voice resounds in speech or song.

This new type of lyre has begun to permeate the musical civilisation of our present time.

A few months ago, the first authoritative book on this instrument was published in Germany. It has the simple title: *Einführung in das Leierspiel*, which, roughly translated means, *An Introduction to Lyre-playing* or, better still, *How to Play the Lyre*. The author is Edmund Pracht, the musician who first conceived of this new instrument thirty years ago, and who, with the help of his friend the sculptor Lothar Gaertner, built the first lyre in 1926. Since that time, almost 1,400 lyres have been built and have found their way into the hands of many people all over the world, bringing delight through their beautiful tone.

The first lyre went through several stages of metamorphosis, and today there are various types, from the big double-bass lyre to the small lyre for children, the latter having only a few strings. All the many different types of lyres can be combined into an orchestra and perform varied kinds of music. A number of lyres accompanying a choir give the best possible background for the human voice.

As a solo instrument the lyre has its special place and purpose. It reveals the beauties of a melody in an outstanding way and gives radiant force to musical phrases.

During the past thirty years, the lyre has become a faithful companion to curative educational work. There are hardly any schools for disabled children based on the principles of Rudolf Steiner in which the lyre does not play an important part in curative work. The lyre accompanies morning and evening song; it is played at the end of the Sunday services, and choir singing is interwoven with lyre playing for all the festivals. In the treatment of deaf children the lyre has proved to be of the greatest help. Many teachers choose to have the lyre as an accompaniment for eurythmical exercises. Restless children are quietened by the sound of the lyre, and sleeping children are awakened by its clear tones in the morning. The lyre is, indeed, an intimate and beloved friend of the curative teacher.

In his book Mr Pracht gives us an introduction to the art of lyre-playing, but it is more than simple advice given on how to play his instrument. It is an introduction to the appreciation of music with lyre playing as a basis. Anybody can learn to play the lyre and, in so doing, draw near to the fountainhead of musical experience, even those who have never learned to read music. All the fundamentals of music are touched upon in this book. Mr Pracht speaks about rhythm and melody, about the intervals and the different keys, the scale, the difference between minor and major, and on every one of these themes he has something new to say, and largely very revealing.

Every statement is explained by musical examples, and the pupil is led, step by step, along the path towards the understanding and performing of music. The book begins with rather simple exercises and goes on to more complicated ones that in the end enable the diligent pupil to perform a great variety of pieces of music on the instrument. Almost anyone who is willing can become an accomplished lyre player.

Those who faithfully pursue the contents of this book will emerge as musicians. They will not only be able to play the lyre, but they will have acquired a fundamental connection to music itself; to that music which reveals itself to a peaceful mind and a quiet heart.

In the opening chapter Mr Pracht says:

> In playing and practising the lyre, we experience the enigma, which even for the human being of this present age, is enshrined in each single tone. We feel called upon to search for the spiritual well of this enigma.[2]

This is one of the principal characteristics of the lyre.

If it were possible that from now on, with the help and guidance of this little book, thousands of people would learn to play the lyre, a great amount of healing power would awaken in the world. How peaceful and creative would people become if, after a day of haste and hard work, instead of settling down to the noise of the wireless and television, they would pick up a lyre and play it, and listen to the eternal voice that speaks though all true music! Their spirits would be filled with new strength and equanimity, and beauty would stir anew in them.

It is my ardent hope that *Einführung in das Leierspiel* will soon be translated into many languages so that it can make its way into all parts of the world. It is a book that can bring spiritual joy to many people. There is no instrument other than the lyre that brings its player so near the fountainhead of true music, and the technique of playing it is not a stumbling block to those who make a regular effort to learn it.

Mr Pracht's book is a guide to the spheres from which music originates, and in writing it, he has set himself and his instrument a worthy monument.

Research

Music Therapy for Deaf and Hearing-Impaired Children

From *The Superintendent's Report: The Camphill Rudolf Steiner Schools for Children in Need of Special Care, 1952–55*

In the last but one report, which was issued in 1949, I mentioned that the training of deaf children using music, sound and speech was introduced in our schools. It was at this time a great new venture, and we can look back now on a task that, without interruption, has continued for almost seven years.

The auditory method is not a new one. It was used time and again in Austria, France and America, but was seldom pursued with enough persistence. Only now is this kind of training coming to the fore again, with several clinics and schools for deaf people adopting this method in the last few years. The use of modern hearing aids has brought this method a great step forwards.

In Camphill, however, our method of auditory training differs from that usually used today. The first and foremost difference is the type of child to whom it is to be applied. Our children are not only partially deaf but disabled in other ways too. They may be blind and deaf, deaf and paralysed, deaf and maladjusted, or deaf and post-encephalitic, and so on. Apart from this difference, we hardly ever use hearing aids, which only in very special circumstances appear to be beneficial to our children.

Our special approach to the use of the auditory method started with two children who were sent to us by their respective Education Authorities. One was a small girl who came with the diagnosis of 'mental retardation and aphasia' (the inability to speak), and the other a boy who was diagnosed as 'ineducable due to severe mental defect'. The boy was even certified and as such was admitted to Camphill. A few weeks' observation revealed that both children were partially deaf. Both were rather clever, made themselves understood by gestures, and tried through lip-reading to understand what was spoken to them. Both had great practical gifts: the girl in housework, the boy in the garden, and they were almost of the same age, around seven years old, when they arrived.

Yet there was a vast difference between them. The girl was slow in her movements, puffy in appearance and somewhat suspicious and restrained. She was shy and blushed a great deal. The boy, on the other hand, was quick, vivacious and full of mischief. He had some difficulties in controlling his movements, which showed definite signs of an athetoid pattern. The girl was fair of complexion, the boy dark. I describe them in such detail, because destiny has been kind in sending us these two children in order to help us find the clue on our way in auditory training.

Here were two children who had an almost equal degree of deafness but were opposites in their behaviour and in their mental as well as physical make-up. We would not have been able to learn the lessons they presented us with were we not familiar with Rudolf Steiner's remarks about the physiology and psychology of hearing. As our observations soon proved, these two children were the most perfect examples of these indications.

Rudolf Steiner has shown us the intimate connection that exists between the functions 'to hear' and 'to move'.

In several of his lectures, he indicated that 'to hear' needs complete silence in the region of the head, and harmonious and active mobility in the sphere of the limbs. Only when this has, to a certain degree, been achieved, can hearing take place. The balance between the upper quiet and the lower mobile poles is brought about by the equilibrium between inhaling and exhaling.

In our two children we had these opposites before us. The boy was so mobile and quick and restless that his head was never at peace; therefore, the quality of listening could not unfold in him. The girl, on the other hand, was so slow and heavy that, to begin with, her movements were few and rather awkward. She had too much of the listening attitude; therefore, she was unable to hear properly. We might also say that she seemed 'to be asleep within the sphere of listening'.

If these two children had not had an auditory obstacle so that their organ of hearing functioned perfectly well, they would have presented the following picture: the girl would have presented as an apathetic child, shy, yet within normal boundaries, whereas the boy would have been a mischievous little youngster, never listening to what he was told yet well able to hear what he wanted to.

I mention this possibility, because it gives us a first understanding of the fact that 'to hear' is not only a matter of the function of the ear as an organ. 'To hear' is a matter for the whole human being who, in their physical, mental and spiritual make-up, has the foundations for this most complicated function. It is therefore necessary to treat and to train the whole human being when dealing with deafness.

A deaf child, indeed, any deaf person, never suffers from a simple, single complaint, and so treatment must be a very individual one. To put a hearing aid into the ears and then think that the main job is done is as wrong as simply to teach a deaf child to lip-read and leave their whole condition as a human being unattended.

Even if these two children whom I have described had had a 'normal' ear organisation, they would have been hard of hearing on account of their personalities. And it was the approach to their individual personalities that, to begin with, was the most important point for us. Here curative education had to be used, with the aim of enlivening the apathetic girl and making the over-active boy quiet.

Both children were very co-operative, and it was a great joy to work with them. We began (and have since done this with every deaf and partially deaf pupil) from two sides: from the side of mobility as well as from the side of listening. The girl's limbs had to be activated, the boy's pacified. Here we found eurythmy was a great help. It had a harmonising effect on the boy's distracted mobility. This again was not simply a process that gave harmony to the limbs. Rather, we observed how the boy, by learning to control his limbs, at the same time developed his ability to listen, which, until then, had been practically nil. The girl, in becoming more active, awakened to the sphere of listening and, for the first time, became interested in observing other people and in 'hearing' what they said.

Along with these eurythmic exercises the teacher sang directly into the ears of the children accompanied by the lyre. The scale was sung in connection with special vowels, thus training the child to hear not only a particular pitch but also the respective vowels. It took only a few weeks before both children reacted satisfactorily. These exercises were done in a semi-darkened room daily for about half an hour. Gradually, the children learned the art of listening, and the acquisition of this quality became a strong incentive for the use of speech.

In a similar way, as the harmonising of their mobility was working upwards and helping them to learn how to hear, so the quality of listening worked, as it were, downwards, and influenced their willingness to speak. It was wonderful to observe how, month after month, the children became more harmonious beings. It dawned on us that the whole human frame was like a musical instrument upon which the human soul plays. Every movement, every spoken word, every gesture, is nothing but the result of the soul playing on the instrument of the body. We also learned by these observations that 'to hear' is not simply brought about by the functioning ear, but here again the whole body and soul is involved. We discovered that Rudolf Steiner's indications were right when he explained that musical rhythm was 'heard' with the limbs, musical harmony experienced with the heart and lungs, and only the melody perceived by the ear-organisation itself.[1]

Thus, all the hearing-music-speech activity in human beings is the result of two complicated processes working together: the process of movement on the one side, and the process of listening on the other. All this must be taken into account when working with deaf children; to approach the problem from one side only is futile. So far, working with deaf children's mobility has been much too much overlooked.

Gradually we learned to see that our two children represented the two main types to be found among deaf people. We also discovered that, in the active type, we had to start with high notes and gradually descend through the scale. The use of the minor key was especially beneficial. For the more passive type, it was necessary to start with low tones and work up through the scale. The use of the major key was important.

After some time, the children began to learn to sing together with their teachers. They learned to understand the spoken word, often without the help of lip-reading.

Soon after the starting with the children, we also made a discovery that was of great importance in working with deaf children. To one degree or another they all have an underdeveloped emotional life. They know the rough emotions of anger and anxiety, fear and shame, but the subtleties of human feelings are a closed realm to them. Here, too, training has to set in. Stories and fairy tales are told, and deaf children learn to express in gestures the emotions of the various characters.

All this takes years of continuous and unbroken effort, and it is important not to lose patience and endurance. One of the obstacles faced by deaf and hard-of-hearing children is their difficulty for remembering sounds and words. Every day they are told certain things, and everything they have learned on one day they have forgotten the next. Many of them substitute their memory for sounds by memory for sight and thereby remember written letters and written words because they can see them. But the spoken word, the melody of vowels and consonants, continuously disappear into oblivion. This is probably the innermost core of deafness in children; that their memory for sounds is deeply disturbed or almost lacking. This can only be built up by the patient diligence and perseverance of the teacher.

The results we have so far achieved are encouraging. We found the best improvements with those children in whom a basic transformation of personality was achieved. When the turmoil of continuous restlessness gradually gives way to calmness and consideration, or when apathy and listlessness becomes transformed into initiative, the main battle was won. It was, however, always easier to perform the first task than the second.

One thing I know for certain. Deafness in children, whatever their other developmental difficulties, can be treated actively, and sometimes this leads to astonishing results. In the training of deaf children, the approach from the side of mobility is as important as the approach from that of listening. Speech has two sides: a motor one and a sensory one. The motor part of their speech must be trained by harmonising the movements of the limbs; at the same time, the sensory part must be trained from the side of the ear. Only by working in this way can better results be achieved.

Deafness in Children: The Ability to Hear and Tumour Formation

Published in *Beiträge zur Erweiterung der Heilkunst* [Contributions to Furthering the Art of Healing], September 1952.

During the past few years I have occupied myself intensively with the issue of deafness in children. Initially I did not intend to publish my findings in relation to this work as it seemed to be a specialised issue. However, it gradually became clear that a number of general medical questions are linked with it and for this reason I decided that it was justified to present some of these findings to a wider group of physicians.

I

In the first issue of *Beiträge zu einer Erweiterung der Heilkunst* [Contributions to Furthering the Art of Healing] (No. 1/2, 1950), Dr Zur Linden pointed to a thesis by Wolfgang Thiele,[1] whose audiometric tests carried out on sixty cancer patients, none of whom had received radiation therapy or been operated upon, showed hearing that was considerably more sensitive than the average found in healthy people. This was, as far as I know, the first time that a link between the ability to hear and cancer had been shown.

Rudolf Steiner gave the following indications in the first doctors' course in connection with this:

> If we consider people who are born deaf and people who have become deaf, it is possible to again make very interesting observations, and more profound associations in nature are revealed. Take note of the following example. As early as childhood, the congenitally deaf would have been predisposed to the worst sorts of tumour formation if they had not been born deaf. This is another one of the natural aids created by nature and it points beyond what can be understood as the individual human organization between birth and death to an influence that intervenes in repeated earthly lives, because that is where it is balanced out. If we trace such phenomena to a certain extent, we reach a point where we begin to grasp the reality of repeated earthly lives.[2]

From totally different sources we thus have here two indications, both of which attempt to describe the same thing. The scientist points out that in a number of people suffering with cancer who had been examined, an enhanced ability to hear was found in comparison to people in a normal state. The spiritual scientist explained that deafness, be it hereditary or acquired, prevented the outbreak of the cancer which was present as a predisposition.

These are two results that seem to complement one another, and it will be necessary to study these indications more closely to understand them. On several occasions Rudolf Steiner tried to establish the close link between ear and tumour formation, and he gave definitive indications about this in the lecture from which the above quotation was taken. There he discusses the connection between the formation of the ear and that of tumours:

Once again, spiritual science is tremendously informative
with regard to this second aspect of the human
organization. It tells us that all the forces that shape
the human ear lie on the same path as the forces that
ultimately lead to internal tumour formation if they
go too far. Our ear formation is the result of a process
that is normalized by holding back the tumour-forming
force at the right stage. The ear is an internal tumour
in the human being, but is kept within normal limits ...
Similarly, the tumour-forming or proliferative process
is significant in the natural world if it takes place at the
correct speed. If you were to do away with this process
not a creature in the world would be able to hear. If
you give it the wrong speed, however, you end up
with everything that takes place in the development of
myomas, carcinomas, and sarcomas.[3]

So here the process of forming the ear, which ultimately
makes the ability to hear possible, is more or less equated
with the tumour-forming process, with the exception that
the latter has been shifted in an abnormal way in space
and time. According to the spiritual scientist, if this shift
in space and time takes place in childhood it will bring
about deafness, which now, in turn, counteracts tumour
formation in the present as a predisposition.

It would be interesting to follow up on this predisposition,
because if this tumour formation in deaf children could be
proven there could be a possibility to trace back the entire
formation of this process a little more precisely.

In Ehrenfried Pfeiffer's crystallisation method we
have a possibility to study the details of processes in the
organism more closely, and last year I instigated thorough
investigations into this in our laboratory. Nine children
whose deafness have different causes were examined and

the results will be reported on shortly. They may give a deeper insight into the whole issue we are discussing here.

II

We will first introduce the nine children and give further details about the degree and nature of their deafness. They will be presented in order of age and referred to by a letter of the alphabet.

Child A

A girl, born on December 11, 1944, in India. The father is from India, the mother from England. The girl is the second child; the sister, who is two years older, developed without hearing problems. There is no indication of deafness in the families of either parent, and the parents themselves have no disabilities. The birth was long but without complications. The child sat up at the age of one and only learned to walk when she was two. The girl's parents gradually began to notice that she did not react to noise, that she dragged her foot when walking, and that she did not use her right hand to pick things up.

When the girl was admitted to us in 1949 she showed a pronounced hemiplegia of the right-hand side, holding her toes in a pointed-foot opposition. The ability to hear was not developed. The girl was restless, showed strong signs of diminished concentration, and only expressed herself through guttural sounds. She displayed a practical intelligence that continued to develop well.

The girl's deafness seems to have a central origin, most likely the same one as the hemiplegia. Bleeding in the mid-brain may well have damaged the acoustic centre so badly that degeneration occurred afterwards.

Child B

A boy, born on the Orkney Isles on January 5, 1941. He is the third child. His sister, who is three years older, is deaf and only learned to speak a few words. His brother, who is one year older than B., has no developmental difficulties. Just before the birth the boy's mother suddenly developed high blood-pressure and B. was born during eclamptic spasms. The mother admitted that his deaf sister had also been born under similar circumstances, while the brother, who had healthy hearing, had a normal birth.

B. was able to sit up at five months and learned to walk at ten months. He never spoke and did not react to noise or tones. He became more restless as he grew older. He had great difficulties falling asleep and displayed an outspoken, destructive tendency. After having spent some time at a school for children with hearing difficulties, he was dismissed because he was unable to fit into the class and was disturbing others due to his continuous restlessness.

B. was brought to us in September, 1949. At that time his restlessness, his destructive tendencies and his crying fits were great. He gradually calmed down, however, and after a year he became a strikingly quiet, peaceful and accessible child. Now he sometimes displays strong tendencies towards melancholy. His deafness is profound and so far has not shown any improvement in spite of extensive special treatment.

As there was no obvious deafness in the family, apart from that of the sister, it might be a case of central damage, perhaps caused by the eclamptic spasms experienced by his mother during the birth.

Child C

A boy born on November 9, 1940, in a town in the middle of England. There is no mention of his parents' ages, nor of any historical details relating to the immediate family. His birth was said to be normal and he developed well until about the sixth month when he had a severe bout of scarlet fever. After this it was assumed that he had become deaf.

As a small child he was extremely restless and prone to severe temper tantrums. At the age of three he was referred to a sanatorium, but whilst he was there he showed signs of good intelligence and so was sent to a school for deaf children. However, because his teachers were unable to deal with his disruptive and undisciplined behaviour, he was admitted to a psychiatric clinic.

In January 1949 he was brought to us. His urge to destroy things was at first unstoppable. He had problems falling asleep and his restlessness was so great that he had to be kept under constant control by an assistant. He displayed a kind of devilish intelligence which he tried to use wherever he could cause damage.

Over the next two years he began to calm down and fit into the social structure of his surroundings. He is now disciplined and has learned basic reading and writing, and the special approach to his deafness achieved good results: he has the first signs of word formation and his ability to hear is much better than before.

He is a deaf child with no clear cause for his deafness. It could be assumed that it had occurred after scarlet fever, and as the middle ear does not show any pathological symptoms it may be assumed that here we are dealing with a degeneration of the organ of Corti after a process of inflammation.

Child D

A boy, born on October 6, 1940, in the south of England. His parents are healthy and two younger siblings developed normally.

In the third month of pregnancy the mother had rubella, yet the birth was without complications. He developed very slowly as a baby, not sitting up until after one year and learning to walk only at the age of two. He never spoke. He was educated in a school for deaf children but was soon dismissed because he was unresponsive and did not take part in the lessons and his environment.

He was admitted to us in September 1950. He is a well-developed child with sharp facial features and deep-set eyes. He was non-speaking, did not take part in anything, and had little urge to move. He appeared not only to be deaf but also to have severe vision problems. He seemed at first totally locked into himself and did not want to take part in his surroundings. He had problems getting to sleep and in the course of a year he developed states of excitement in which he started to self-harm: he would hit his head against hard objects and beat his fist into his face. At the same time, however, he became more approachable and more dependent on his carer, but he remains mute without any sign of articulation.

This is a deaf child whose deafness almost certainly is the result of a developmental disturbance of the inner ear due to rubella.

Child E

A boy, born in the north of Scotland on September 29, 1939. He is the second child and has a three-year older brother who has no developmental difficulties. The pregnancy was without complications and so was the birth. As a baby Child E developed slowly, learning to sit up at one year and to walk at eighteen months.

He never learned to speak and was examined by various physicians, as it was not obvious whether he was deaf or had a learning disability. He was restless, unable to concentrate and aimless in his activities. When he was five years old he was diagnosed with a learning disability and the diagnosis 'deaf-mute' was dropped.

At the age of nine he was admitted to us. He was frail and thin for his age, with a pointed face and an empty look on his face. He was anxious and on the run all the time, and it took quite a while before he gained a little trust and confidence. He sometimes made an effort to speak but was unable to vocalise at all.

After many months' observation it became clear that he was deaf, with other senses somewhat stunted in their development as a result. We then worked on the diagnosis 'deaf based on pre-and post-natal traumas'. We have as yet not been able to determine the nature of the traumas.

Child F

A girl, born in the middle of Scotland on April 6, 1939, the only child of seemingly healthy parents. The birth was normal, though a month premature. The baby was breastfed for a month, but then began to lose weight and had to be admitted to hospital. F. remained there for two months and developed quite well from then onwards. She was able to sit up at one year and began to walk at eighteen months. She never learned to speak and was an unruly and stubborn child. At five years old she was examined by a specialist and diagnosed with sensory aphasia. Hearing tests were not done in this examination according to the precise report we have. The child was admitted to our school in December 1945 with this diagnosis. Soon after her admission the diagnosis could be established as deafness. The child neither reacted to tones nor to loud or soft noises, but because of her intelligence she learned the art of lip-reading and thus managed to produce some muffled words.

She responded very well to the exercises for deafness and

also learned to speak. Our diagnosis was fully confirmed in the examination done by a specialist last year.

There is no doubt that this girl had a congenital condition.

Child G

A boy born in the north of Scotland on March 17, 1939. Two older sisters developed normally. Like Child F. he was born one month early, and the birth was complicated by a breech-position. He developed slowly and only sat up at one year. He began to walk at the age of two and his gait was unsure for a long time. There were no signs of any speech development. When he was two years old he suddenly had haemorrhages over the whole of his body and was in hospital for some time.

He then went to a kindergarten, where he was very restless and did not make any progress in his speech development. He was diagnosed with a learning disability.

He was admitted to us in April 1946. After a more thorough investigation and observation it appeared that the child's entire movement organisation was disturbed. He displayed outspoken athetotic movements, an unstable gait and a lack of word understanding. Hearing tests showed a very much reduced ability to hear, although his intelligence was good and most likely above average with a good ability to concentrate and to grasp things.

All these symptoms showed quite clearly that the picture he displayed had been caused by an underlying disturbance, which can also be seen as the result of nuclear jaundice. There must have been a severe brittleness of the vascular walls that during the complicated birth may well have led to bleeding in the midbrain, which governs the toning functions of the skeletal muscles, as well as to bleeding in the neighbouring acoustic centre. The child made amazing progress, learned to speak and hear and may be designated as normal in his academic and other achievements.

Our diagnosis was deafness caused by bleeding on the midbrain combined with athetosis.

Child H

A girl, born September 5, 1938, in a small town in the north of England. The second of four children born to a single mother with learning difficulties who is at present living in an institution. Child H. grew up with her grandmother in extremely poor circumstances. She learned to walk at twenty-one months, but never learned to speak. At age five she went to a school for deaf children but resisted all attempts to educate her. She displayed no ability to grasp things, although her intelligence was average. She remained in this school for six years and was then dismissed.

In November 1951 she was admitted to us, and the observation and examination process presented a very complicated picture of her illness. Her word understanding is totally blocked and she reacts only to her first name. She does not react to tones, music or noises. She has some practical understanding, is quite stubborn and very undeveloped in her feeling life. Nevertheless, Child H. is a charming and lively little girl.

There is no doubt that, apart from a total lack of word understanding, there is a certain degree of deafness. So far it has not been possible to determine the cause of the deafness.

Child I

A boy, born on November 11, 1933, in the south of England. He is the fourth child, with two brothers and a sister whose circumstances are unknown. His mother loves children;

she is deaf and lives separated from her husband because he keeps on getting into trouble with the law and often spends time in prison because of deception and fraud. Until the age of five Child I. lived with his mother but was then taken into care in a large care organisation. He learned to speak with some difficulty, and it was soon discovered that he was deaf. He was then educated in various institutions for deaf people without much success.

He came to us in April 1948. His academic knowledge was very much delayed. He was able to write a little but could not do sums; his reading was elementary. His speech was slurred and inarticulate and his words rather primitive. He was short-sighted, slow, obstinate and quite withdrawn.

Further examination showed signs of congenital hypothyroidism with his deafness a symptom of the whole syndrome. He has improved quite a lot over the past few years. His ability to hear is better and his speech more articulated.

So we are dealing here with children and young people between the ages of seven and eighteen, who could be designated as more or less hard of hearing or deaf. The degree of deafness varies as does its origin. It accords with my long experience that every deaf child demands a special study so as to find out the degree and type of deafness. I am of the opinion that there are no two deaf children in whom the same form of deafness is present.

Blood tests were done on these nine children according to Ehrenfried Pfeiffer's crystallisation method, with six plates produced for each child. For the sake of an easier overview a short description of how the plates have been divided up in their different areas will be presented in advance of the report on the results.

The plates are divided as shown in the numbered circle (I) in the diagram. The head zone is within the half circle that spans fields 10 and 11. Fields 9 and 12 rarely show disturbances belonging to the head. The lung zone is in fields 6 and 7. The heart shapes are mainly located in field 6 and often stretch over into 5. In field 4 there can be seen liver disorders, which often radiate out into fields 3 and 8. The kidney points lie in fields 2 and 3. If there are disturbances in the kidney zone, forms will radiate from these points right into the periphery of these fields, but also sometimes into the peripheries of fields 1 and 4. Bladder disorders – fields 2 and 3 – are visible in the middle axis to the head zone of the picture.

The kidney disorders visible in the pictures of deaf children are sometimes situated comparatively near to the periphery and also reach over into fields 1 and 4. Nevertheless it can be determined with certainty that we are here dealing with the kidney area and not with the gonads, which sometimes take up this position. The point of gravity has been marked and only the centres of the disturbance have been marked in.

The following results could be derived from the blood-crystal images.

Child A: blood crystal image of September 25, 1951 (II)

From the kidney points, which lie on the borders of the second and third up to the sixth and seventh fields radiating shapes go into the periphery of fields 1, 2, 3, and 4: between both forms there is the shape of a bubble. All three of the disturbed forms are accompanied and interspersed by large signs of carcinoma. In field 11 and on some plates, and also as a trace in field 10, there lies a narrow, pointed oval, the shape of an ear. These shapes are also accompanied by signs of carcinoma, although not very clearly.

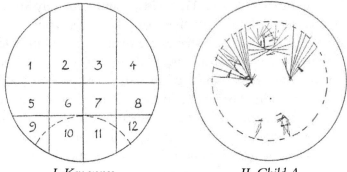

I. Key zones   II. Child A

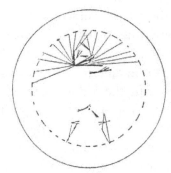

III. Child B

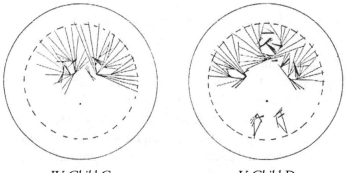

IV. Child C   V. Child D

Blood crystalisation plates 1 (1952)

146

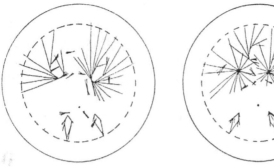

VI. Child E   VII. Child F

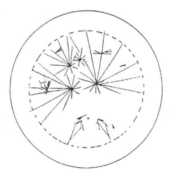

VIII. Child G

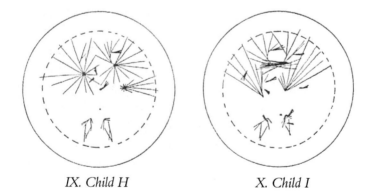

IX. Child H   X. Child I

Blood crystalisation plates 2 (1952)

Child B: blood crystal image of July 27, 1950 (III)

The picture shows the dark-blue-green spots or streaks often found in images of pre-cancerous patients. Three of the six images show a bubble shape, which includes signs of carcinoma, and in the other three there is one with a shape indicating a fibrotic irritation at the upright middle axis between fields 2 and 3. The head zone shows vague, earlike shapes and signs of carcinoma.

Child C: blood crystal image of August 22,1951 (IV)

This picture has already been earmarked by its colour and structure as a so-called 'kidney-image'. Both in fields 2 and 3 there lies a form of a swelling. These forms are spreading to fields 1 and 4. Next to these forms there are one or two clear signs of carcinoma. One would have to speak in this case about tumour-forming processes with the tendency to malignancy. No ear-like shapes have been pictured.

Child D: blood crystal image of September 18, 1959 (V)

The image with its blue-green colour is similar to the one of Child B.; it is also permeated by dark flecks. In fields 2 and 3 there lies the basis of a form of a swelling. These forms are drawing towards fields 1 and 4. Below the forms in fields 2 and 3, spreading out up to fields 6 and 7, there are signs of carcinoma. Bedded in between both tumour shapes and pushing them aside is a bubble-like form that has within it signs of carcinoma. The head-area shows up earlike shapes on the base of which there are also small signs of carcinoma. The image may be compared with one of a patient who is in an advanced stage of cancer.

Child E: blood crystal image of April 30, 1951 (VI)

This image can be described with almost the same words as the previous one. It has the same blue-green colour, but the dark fields are less prominent. A similar form of a swelling lies in fields 2 and 3 and spreads out towards fields 1 and 4. On some plates they have their starting point at the border to fields 6 and 7 and extend to the periphery. These forms are surrounded and permeated by smaller and larger signs of carcinoma. The bladder-form is missing here. The head zone indicates clear narrow oval shapes, which are also joined on both sides by signs of carcinoma.

Child F: blood crystal image of May 22, 1951 (VII)

As was the case with children B., D., and E., the image of this child is also blue-green with dark flecks. The kidneys are marked by shapes of inflammation with their centre in fields 2 and 3, covering fields 1 and 4, and also radiating out to fields 5 and 8. A bubble shape that is lying in between them has been indicated only fleetingly on some plates as they have been stopped from developing by the expanding inflammation shapes. On the rest of the plates the bubble-form fills fields 2 and 3, pressing the inflammation shapes out towards fields 1 and 4 (an attempt has been made in this particular illustration to unite both kinds of images). The signs of inflammation, which are often incomplete, are permeated as well as surrounded by signs indicating carcinoma.

In the head zone there are narrow ovals with earlike shapes. Due to the contradiction that is formed by signs of inflammation and cancer the image of a Viscum reaction may be rejected.

Child G: blood crystal image of September 7, 1950 (VIII)

The crystallisation shows a lot of yellow-green things. It is in this respect similar to the image of Child C. In fields 2 and 3 there are signs of inflammation, which can be assigned to the kidneys and the bladder. They radiate out towards the periphery of fields 1 and 4 and reach all the way to fields 5 and 8. Individual small signs of carcinoma are spread over the entire image. In the head zone some earlike shapes are pictured.

Child H: blood crystal image of December 11, 1951 (IX)

The colour of this image is blue-green with yellow-green streaks shooting through it, especially in the centre of the image. In fields 2 and 3 there are signs of inflammation, which radiate out to fields 1 and 4. At the crossing point of fields 3, 4, and 7 there is again a shape indicating inflammation. It belongs to the area of the liver. Clearly pronounced ovals with earlike shapes in the head zone can be found on three plates, and on the remaining three plates there were only vague indications of them. Next to the forms of inflammation and permeating these there can clearly be seen small signs of carcinoma. This image may be compared with a case of a kidney infection in a precancerous state.

Child I: blood crystal image of March 22, 1951 (X)

This image has a blue-green colour and shows up dark flecks or streaks similar to the ones described in the reports for children B., D., E. and F. From points at the lower edge of fields 2 and 3, fan-formed bundles of crystal radiate out into the periphery; on two of the six plates they are situated in fields 6 and 7. Between both these forms at the upper end of the vertical middle axis there lies a bubble shape, which is permeated by signs of carcinoma. Such signs are also connected with the kidney-shapes, and with the narrow ovals of the head zone.

All the images that were made of deaf children show signs of carcinoma, and almost exclusively in connection with kidney and ear shapes.[4]

III

Although the indication by Rudolf Steiner quoted in the first part of this essay could be confirmed by the results reported in the second part, not much has been achieved towards the clarification and explanation of these facts themselves. The question is: by what means and why is it possible that a certain degree of congenital or acquired deafness can prevent cancer? This question is closely linked with the connection between the tumour-forming process and the formation of the ear as indicated by Steiner. Is it possible to find an answer already today?

I have the impression that very profound problems of organic and human existence are hidden behind this indication, and I will attempt to give some hints that might in future lead us closer to the answer aimed for. A more fulsome answer would be an essential contribution to the problem of tumour formation as such, but we are still quite far away from this. In spite of Gisbert Husemann's foundational work in which the parts of the problem were shown in a wider overview, we are still at the beginning.[5] The following explanations might take us a small step further.

If one follows up on the formation of the ear in the comparative anatomy of animals, already after a superficial study the following facts become clear: namely that an ear-like organ only begins to form where a lung comes about as an organ for breathing. Although all gill-breathing animals have an organ for equilibrium, and possibly also an organ for sensing noise (the utricle and saccule), it is only when a lung has been formed that the first beginnings of the organ of Corti come about in the form of the lagena. This is an extension of the saccule in some vertebrates and corresponds to the cochlear duct in mammals.

For this reason the development of the lung has to be placed parallel to the formation of the inner ear. There are, however, indications given by Steiner where he speaks about the true process of lung formation in the human organism. He describes the spheres surrounding the earth that lie beyond the warmth mantle of the planet, and then, from within outwards, there follow the spheres of the light, chemical and life ethers. Rudolf Steiner literally says at this point:

> But the formation of the solid earth also has its
> counterpart in the cosmos. And this counterpart, you see,
> is the formation of life, the origin of vitalisation. Actually,
> this counterpart is what is to be found in the life forces
> themselves. These, therefore, come from even farther
> away than the chemical forces and are totally killed off
> within the solid element in external, nonhuman nature
> ... Our Earth would be subject to constant proliferation
> of life, to the constant development of carcinomas, if this
> proliferation of extra-telluric factors were not countered
> by the mercurial process, by the effects that Mercury
> exerts on the Earth. It is important to at least think about
> these issues for once. In oyster shell formation, what
> generally takes place on the formation of the solid earth
> – which we can also call the formative element in the
> process of becoming substance – is held back at an earlier
> stage. Oyster shell is prevented from being completely

subsumed by the earth-forming process only because it still has connections to the ocean, to the water. It is held back and solidifies at an earlier stage in the earth-forming process.[6]

Within these indications lie some mysteries of creation because what has here been described as a 'mercurial process' appears in the human organism as the lung. This is why Rudolf Steiner then goes on to describe the two 'different aspects' of the lungs:

> First, they are the respiratory organs. But as strange as it may sound, this is the situation only on a superficial level. At the same time, they are also regulatory organs for the earth-forming process deep within the human being. If we ... study the process that forms the lungs in an inner sense we find that they are the opposite of the activity expressed in oyster shell formation. In its lung-forming process, the human organisation has incorporated a process that lies above the zone of chemistry in the external universe ... You must look for pulmonary degeneration in processes similar to those that appear in oyster shell formation or the like and certainly also in the formation of snail shells, and so on.[7]

Now, it is exactly the formation of the snail shell that occurs in the building of the organ of Corti, which is closely connected with the forming of the lung as we were able to show above. Something therefore happens within the human organism that used to take place in the course of the evolution of the earth outside, because, as Steiner says prior to this:

> [The] oyster shell is prevented from being completely subsumed by the earth-forming process only because it

still has connections to the ocean, to the water. It is held
back and solidifies at an earlier stage in the earth-forming
process.[8]

It is the same for the organ of Corti because it retains
its connection to the sea, the cerebrospinal fluid, to water,
to the endolymph, and thus retains an earlier stage within
itself. Yet because the formation of the organ of Corti
retains an earlier stage of the earth within itself, the forces
that would otherwise be within it are being held back.
These, however, are the forces that form tumours, which
are being held back in their rightful place.

The following thoughts could arise from this. The
Mercury process residing in the lung continually regulates
the forces of earth-formation and solidification that occur
inside the human organism. In the lung are contained
those formative life forces that outside in the cosmos form
the outermost layer of the earth-mantle and all the time
want to lead to cancerous tumour formations. The fact that
this does not happen can be attributed to the hardening
Mercury forces, which are active both outside and within
the human corporeality.

So it seems that the organ of the lung is the training
centre for all the tumour-forming processes. From here
the forces stream into the periphery of the organism and
are continuously normalised by the forces of the Mercury
sphere that are streaming around.

The formation of the organ of Corti is connected with
this function of the lung. Within it, the tumour-forming
force is not only normalised by the Mercury forces, it is
also being held back at an earlier evolutionary stage of the
earth. This brings about a physical hearing organ instead of
a physical carcinoma.

In connection with this it might be interesting to
point out that the development of air-filled cavities, or

pneumatisation, of the temporal bone starting from the middle ear happens developmentally and formatively like the development of the bronchial tree in the embryo. Here something happens, one stage further on, that is being withheld in the forming of the inner ear. If we follow the pneumatisation of the petrous bone (the pyramid-shaped part of the temporal bone) properly, the impression cannot be avoided that we are dealing with a destructive process in the form of tumour-like swellings that only comes to a halt at the last moment.[9]

From all this it becomes clear that the formation of the ear, and also of the mastoid area, has been induced by the lung. The vesicle of the ear, which is formed out of the ectoderm, is initially only in the position to form the organs of the static apparatus and the sensation of noise. Only gradually is a part of the ear-vesicle drawn into the formation of the lagena and the organ of Corti during the last stage of the phylogeny, but this only happens *after* a lung has been fully developed.[10] This formation has been induced out of the life forces present in the lung, which are really tumour-forming forces. The same forces then lead to the forming of the pneumatic space in the mastoid (jaw) bone.

Yet if we again study the phylogeny and comparative anatomy of the lung it becomes clear that the transformation of the swim bladder of the fish into the lung of the amphibian is being accompanied by the sudden formation of the limbs. As if in an act of creation, the animal that has limbs appears together with a lung that is able to breathe. It is as if the breath-stream being actively drawn inside brings along with it the formation of the limbs. This act of creation is all the time still visible if one studies the transformation of the tadpole into a frog. This demonstrates the double aspect of the lung: upwards it forms the organ of Corti, downwards the limbs.

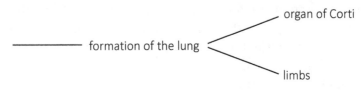

Lung-Corti-limbs

The forming of the limbs is the expression of the forces of the lung that Rudolf Steiner calls 'Mercurial'. At a different place he says about this:

> And what imparts power to our limbs, that enables us to become beings of movement, comes from Mercury.[11]

On another occasions he characterises the Mercury forces in the following way:

> Similar to the moon, Mercury has its target points more in the inner being of man, working from outside only on the human countenance. In the part lying below the region of the heart, its forces are effective by taking hold inwardly of the human organization and, in turn, streaming forth from there. Mercury's chief task is to bring the astral body's activity into all breathing and circulation processes of the human being. Mercury is the intercessor between the astral body and the rhythmic processes in man. Thus, we are able to say that its forces intercede between the astral element and the rhythmic activity. Due to this, similar to the moon forces, the Mercury forces also intervene in the whole human metabolism, but only insofar as the metabolism is subject to rhythm, reacting upon rhythmic activity.[12]

The metabolic processes connected with rhythm, however, are exactly the forces living in the limbs that bring about and maintain mobility. Yet within this are situated the stream of forces that continually lead to the release of the tumour-forming processes, so that the lung gives us both: the tumour-forming force, which is also the force that forms the ear, and the limb-forming rhythmic system, which counteracts the surplus of tumour formation.

Seen from this point of view, however, yet another area comes to light that may be accessible to observation but which has so far not been understood properly, namely that if one has the opportunity in short succession to visit an institute for those who are blind and an institute for those who are deaf, one will be deeply impressed by the opposite atmospheres present there. In the institute for the blind there is utter peace and quiet: it is as if everyone was walking on tiptoes and speaking very softly and quietly. In the place for those who are deaf, on the other hand, everything is loud, noisy and impetuous. A Dionysian-like element lives within the children who are deaf, and their urge to move and the lack of restraint in their motor activity is one of their most striking symptoms. There is no doubt that this urge to move is linked with the fact that their ability to express themselves in speech is completely or partly lacking and that instead of speech the movement of the limbs ensues. Yet this is not the only and most essential reason, because people who become deaf or hard of hearing only in old age, and who then also have problems with speech, do not display the uncontrolled motor activity of deaf children.

Is it perhaps not so that the motor activity carries the forces that have a releasing effect on the tumour-forming forces? The exuberant Mercury in the motor system, which is being counteracted by congenital or acquired deafness, continually brings release to what otherwise wants to establish itself physically as tumour or carcinoma. This is why Ernst Hass writes:

> In a large number of all cancer patients we are dealing
> with people who, both physically and also in relation to
> the most varied physical expressions of life, react slowly
> and sluggishly. The cancerous constitution thus stands in
> direct contrast to the predisposition to inflammation as a
> hypoergic general situation and comes to expression in a
> similar way on all levels of existence.[13]

With this we have come back to the first indications,
which make it clear why deafness in early childhood
prevents the occurrence of terrible tumour-formations;
but also, in contrast to this, that the occurrence of the
carcinoma comes together with a heightened ability to hear.
The ability to hear is always the result of motor activity
that has been brought to rest: listening is only possible if
the urge to move is harmonised and controlled. Yet if this
situation is suddenly turned into a hypoergic one, it will
result in the formation of carcinoma.

In summary, we could therefore say: the tumour-
forming forces originate in the lung; from here, in the
course of phylogeny, they reach the ear-vesicles, form the
lagena and finally the organ of Corti. The Mercury forces,
on the other hand, streaming in from the surroundings, are
intimately related to the lung region and form the limbs
from there. The latter forces could be designated as forces
that prevent tumours. In the way that in deaf children those
forces are especially enhanced through the inability to hear,
they counteract any existing predisposition to carcinoma.
This leads to an initial understanding of the indications
given by Rudolf Steiner in relation to this issue.

Therapeutic Endeavours

Music Therapy Conferences

Camphill and Newton Dee, January 1961 and 1962

According to the lecture index of the Karl König Archives, König gave three lectures on music in January 1961. No notes of these lectures are available, however. At the same time, a music therapy conference had been held. We know from a report that Mrs Schüppel took part in this conference. She described how she travelled more or less in the wake of Paul Nordoff and Clive Robbins when they spent six months in 1960 travelling through Europe collecting various experiences of music therapy in a number of curative-educational institutions. They visited Camphill in June 1960. The music therapy conference, which was held over Christmas and New Year of 1961/62, was covered by journal entries and a report that König prepared afterwards. They are included here, too. Margarethe Reuschle also wrote a report on it, which follows this section (see 'A Music Conference in Camphill').

The Mercury Bath (1961)
Katarina Seeherr

During a music therapy conference in January 1961, of which no notes are available, a special music therapy composition known as the Mercury Bath came about through the collaboration of Karl König and Maria Schüppel. In reply to a question about the origin of the Mercury Bath, Mrs Maria Schüppel said in 1992 that it must have been during the conference in Camphill during Christmas and New Year 1960/61. Every day during this conference she had the opportunity to play a composition in the planetary scale for that day to König. After playing her composition in the D-scale, König said: 'This is a real Mercury Bath; through this one can learn to breathe.' This is how the name 'Mercury Bath' arose. At that time Mrs Schüppel demonstrated her composition on the piano with her left hand playing an octave lower than the right hand. The right hand began, playing the 'I'- octave – the octave above middle C – and then the left hand, the astral octave – below middle C – started in canon one tone later. This original version in 7/8 beat was only played upwards. Maria Schüppel also mentioned the importance of the interplay between the astral- and the 'I'-octaves in the ever-repeating interval sequences of tenth-tenth-eleventh-sixth-sixth-fifth-ninth. A continuous sequence of expansion and contraction thus arises, while the etheric body is being addressed through the continuous alternation of minor and major.[1]

Opposite: Mercury Bath score[2]

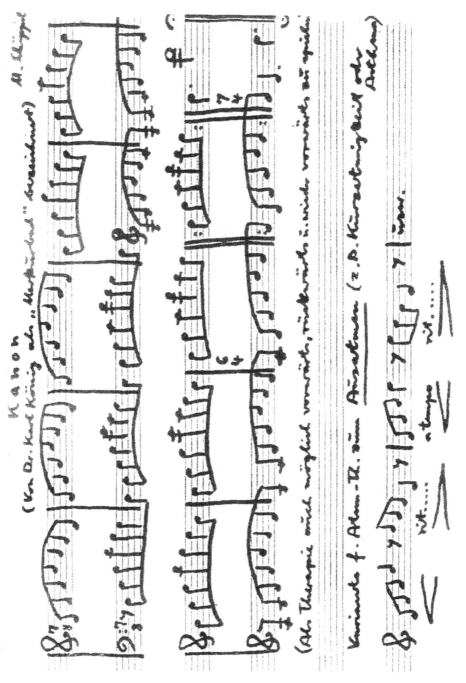

A musical physiology (1962)

Notes from talks about music and singing, January 6, 1962

Breathing

Its origin lies in the sun. It is radiated out from there.

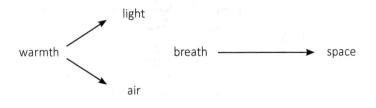

Space emerges when light is formed. The space is filled with air and has thus become breath.

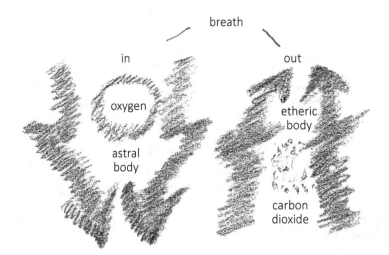

In our time the breath is no longer ensouled. Instead light sends the cosmic spirit via its rays into the human sensory organisation.[3]

The seven life processes originate in breathing:[4]

> Breathing corresponds to the prime.
> Warming corresponds to the second.
> Nourishing corresponds to the third.
> Secretion corresponds to the fourth.
> Maintaining corresponds to the fifth.
> Growing corresponds to the sixth.
> Reproducing corresponds to the seventh.

The scale starts with the *prime*; it shows that it is a breath-filled basic tone from which all that follows originates.

In the *second* this breath is warmed through. Now a kind of personal character begins to show itself. The world is mirrored in the special facets of this scale.

Everything has become fixed in the *third*. As major or minor third substance which is more or less tonal is absorbed and processed in a major or minor mode.

The personality of the scale emerges with the *fourth*. It does not yet reveal itself but is actively separating itself out. It is contracted like a knot.

The manifestation only begins with the *fifth*. Here the personality is gaining form. What had been separated begins to *assert itself*. It begins to appear. This is the music of the fifth.

In the *sixth* growth enters in: enlargement and expansion begin to appear.

In the *seventh* everything is already going beyond itself and becomes something new and different. The process of *reproducing* has been reached. (See figure overleaf.)

As breathing consists of both inhalation and exhalation there are also two groups of organs for it, which are, as it were, created by the breath and now serve it: the *larynx* and the *bladder.*

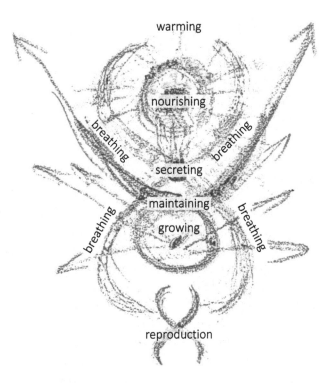

Sketch of the life processes

Anatomy of the larynx

Cricoid cartilage	physical body
Thyroid cartilage	ether body
Arytenoid cartilage	astral body
Epiglottis	'I'
Hyoid (tongue) bone	Manas (spirit self)

A *complete* human being is thus represented here, so it can become the carrier of speech sound.

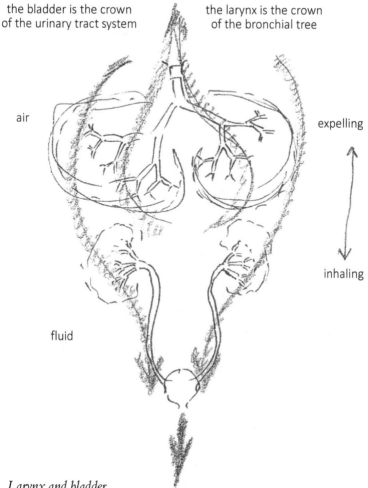

the bladder is the crown
of the urinary tract system

the larynx is the crown
of the bronchial tree

air

expelling

inhaling

fluid

Larynx and bladder

Cricoid cartilage	pelvis
Thyroid cartilage	breast
Arythenoid cartilage	shoulder blades
Epiglottis	skull bone

And there come over the human being the seven from below, the eight from above, the nine from behind, the ten from the foundations of the rocky vault, and the ten from within, while the mother cares for the suckling child.[5]

In the lecture 'Human Expression Through Tone and Word', Rudolf Steiner said:

Song is indeed a genuine remembering – though by earthly means – of that which we experienced during pre-earthly existence. For in our rhythmic system we are much closer to the spiritual world than in our thinking system.[6]

The question arises: Why do only the birds sing? How did it come about that it is precisely they who have the possibility to create a song?

Yet if we study the structure of the bird skeleton the answer reveals itself. The composition of the rump is so that the shoulder blades touch on the pelvis and that the breastbone is enormously developed. The body of the bird thus shows the same morphology that is present in the human larynx.

This shows that the *bird* is a *larynx,* which is the reason why the formation of tone takes place in its entire body.

The epiglottis, however, is the syrinx, the end part of the trachea and the start of the bronchia. They have been arranged within the breast-stomach cavity in the same way as the epiglottis has within the larynx.

The whole bird is therefore larynx and thus the creator of tone.

The bird's neck corresponds to the throat and the head to our oral parts.

The brain of the bird, however, can only be compared with the nerve region, which we call the brain stem, and the corpora quadrigemina with the pineal gland.

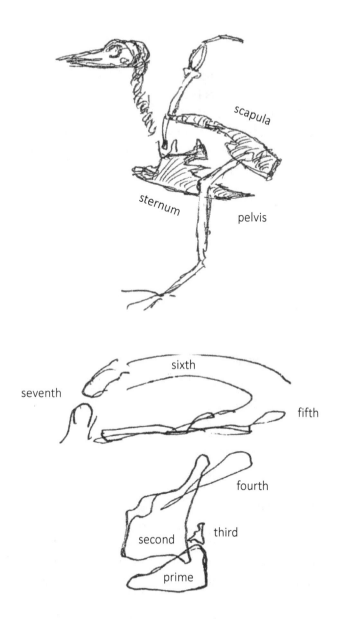

Top: Sketch of a bird skeleton
Bottom: The intervals shaping the tones

The seven life processes

After having gone through all the planetary scales, an image approximately as follows begins to appear.

It first resounds in space of Saturn. There it is like a gentle fire. Gradually, the more voices and counter-voices are heard, the more evident the centres of warmth and fire in each upper arm, in both upper legs and in the hind-head become.

It is something like this:

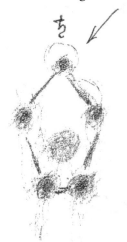

Blood formation

Opposite: The seven life processes
Translation of top part:

♄ (Saturn)	breathing	consuming	(Saturn) ♄
☉ (Sun)	warming	combustion	(Jupiter) ♃
☽ (Moon)	nourishing	sedimentation	(Mars) ♂
♂ (Mars)	secretion	(Sun) ☉	
☿ (Mercury)	maintaining	hardening	(Mercury) ☿
♃ (Jupiter)	growing	maturing	(Venus) ♀
♀ (Venus)	reproducing	generating	(Moon) ☽

Die sieben Lebensprozesse

♄   Atmung . . . . . — . . . Verbrauchen ♄

☉   Wärmung . . . — — . . . Verbrennen ♃

☽   Ernährung . — — — . . Ablagerung ♂

     ♂ Absonderung ☉

☿   Erhaltung . — . — . . . Verhärtung ☿

♃   Wachstum . — — — . . . Reifung ♀

♀   Reproduktion . — — — . . Generation ☽

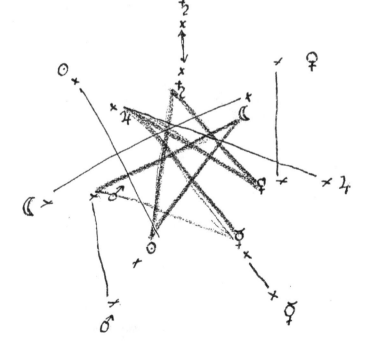

What is this? Are they centres for the formation of blood? All of it is certainly warmth, which is permeating us, but what role does this warmth play which is thus arranged within us? Is it connected with the formation of swellings, such as sarcoma or leukaemia, etc?

It is different with the *Sun scale*. There the stimulus lies below the diaphragm. It is centred around the solar plexus and there is no doubt that both the sympathetic and the para-sympathetic systems are stimulated and experienced by it. Everything is very bright, very harmonising, like streaming light.

A new picture arises with the *Moon scale*. Here everything is centred around the region of the stomach. Now I know why the stomach is moon shaped. This, however, makes the sound of the waxing and the waning moon into an experience. The HCl (hydrochloric) digestion *increases* with the waxing moon and *decreases* with the waning moon. Stomach ulcers are therefore like an imprint of the effects of the full moon.

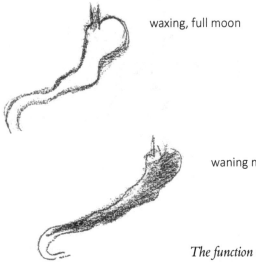

waxing, full moon

waning moon

The function of the stomach depends on the moon

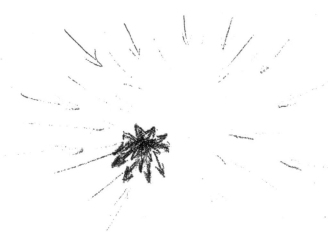

Cosmic iron

The *Mars scale* again presents a totally different experiential picture. When it resounds, certain sensations are stimulated in the environment that could be designated as blood-forming forces. They come from all sides out of the cosmos and are in fact identical with what Rudolf Steiner described as cosmic iron: meteoric iron.

And to the right, in the region of the liver, a centre for secretion is being formed. It is as if poison is being excreted from the building up process. It is very clearly present *on the right.*

Through the *Mercury scale* a totally different picture arises again. It is the scale in which the mirrored form is *exactly* the opposite, thus bringing about a true mirror image. Here we have a sensation of a pearl-like enlivening twinkling. It streams upwards and downwards within the body and cannot be localised; there is hardly any organ that can connect with it. Yet the sensation is stronger below the diaphragm than above it. Everything is, however, stressed *on the left* and the impression may arise that the entire lymph formation takes place here.

In the *Jupiter scale* something very special occurs. Here the forces that form the liver and not the forces that form the blood are very strongly involved in the experience. They are images of alchemical forces that arise and stream into the right-hand side as if coming from spiritual realms (I do not know where they come from). It is as if they are closing in on the liver. At the same time, however, a kind of reflected surface arises in the region of the forehead. This surface is, as it were, lit up, illuminating that which is bound by substance below.

In the *Venus scale* this form of localisation is no longer possible. Everything remains undetermined. Nevertheless, one has the impression that it rises up out of the depths of

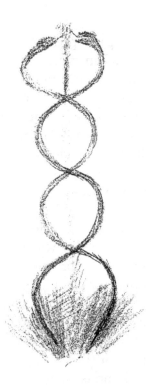

This is will

the body and that we are dealing here with the archetypal sound stream. Like a staff of Mercury it rises upwards and opens up into a point, which may well be described as the region of the brain stem. It is the area of the *corpora quadrigemina* and the epiphysis or pineal gland.

I feel the substance of the world resound in my warmth.[7]

Thus a first attempt of a musical physiology came about. It is connected with Eugen Kolisko,[8] whom we commemorated at the end of the course.

We also experienced that the voice of conscience resounds in the tritone.

Notes from Karl König's Diary

Tuesday, January 2, 1962
In the morning I first dealt with the mail and then I did clay modelling with the musicians. We modelled the larynx. There is much better contact now and a good collaboration is beginning to be established, especially in relation to the interpretations I am able to give of the planetary scales.

Wednesday, January 3, 1962
Now the music conference is continuing. We completed the modelling of the larynx and then I spoke about the metamorphosis of the four cartilages and added them to the structure of the sensory and super-sensory human being. I also spoke about the types of metamorphosis, and it became very lively and impressive.

The preparation for the second lecture about conscience is not easy. But gradually, after including forgetting, misplacing and losing, and also using the lecture on the 'voice of conscience', the threefold image of conscience is beginning to take shape for me. This also flows together with the St John's imagination and thus a wonderful image arises which I will attempt to bring to the friends.

Thursday, January 4, 1962
The riddle of birdsong is taken up again with a lecture by Rudolf Steiner and during the study of the bird skeleton it suddenly becomes clear that the body of the bird is a larynx, the breastbone the thyroid cartilage, the shoulder blade the cricoid cartilage etc. Neck and beak, however, are like the windpipe, tongue and mouth, and thus the whole bird is a producer of tone. This discovery fills me with joy, but it would not be understood were I to present it to the course.

We had a very interesting musical evening provided by our guests. A large number of old and new compositions from Africa and Ireland resounded, as well as many of the planetary scales.

Friday, January 5, 1962
In the morning the music group came together again, and I spoke about the seven life processes and their transformations through the Luciferic and Ahrimanic influences. This showed up quite a few new parallels.

A Music Conference in Camphill

Margarethe Reuschle

From *The Cresset*, Easter, 1962

A certain amount in the field of music therapy has been worked out in Camphill over the years, but in comparison to other treatments it is still only a beginning waiting to be developed. In the last two or three years, Miss Veronika Bay has been working quietly with a small group of Dutch musicians (including especially Mrs Marja Slotemaker de Bruine) according to the indications of the anthroposophical musician Anny von Lange.[1] Miss Bay and her friends wished to spend part of the Christmas holiday in Camphill to report on what they had worked on; they also hoped to hear from Dr König and others in Camphill about their experiences in music therapy. In spite of ice and deep snow, the small party ventured up to Aberdeen bringing with them a musician from Berlin, Maria Schüppel, together with her many instruments.

Although no programme had been made, a way of working was soon found. Every morning at 10 o'clock we met at Murtle House and occupied ourselves with the scales that Anny von Lange had worked out as a foundation for a new development in music in her book *Mensch, Musik und Kosmos* [man, music and cosmos]. These are the familiar modal scales played upwards but sung or played in a mirrored form downwards. According to Rudolf Steiner, every tone in the C-major scale can be assigned to a planet, and so on every day of the week we worked with one of these scales. When two groups sang the scales and their mirrored form against one another the result was the most astonishing chords that seemingly came from distant spheres. It was also impressive to see the interpretation of the different scales in eurythmy as demonstrated by Mrs Reeskamp.

After this first hour we met with Dr König and reported on the work done. Dr König discussed with us the possibilities for therapy that arose out of listening to the new sounds described above, and his indications were to a great extent based on the experiences of Mrs Slotemaker. Then Dr König discussed various physiological aspects that are of importance to musicians and to singers. He dealt, for instance, with breathing, sense physiology, the life processes, and also spoke about those archetypal singers: the birds. It was a wonderful thing then to model the human larynx in coloured wax under his direction.

In the afternoon the group of musicians played for the children in the schools and in the Newton Dee Community. Two evenings were given to the staff of the schools and therapeutic music from ancient and present times was demonstrated. Mrs Slotemaker acquainted us with short pieces of music she had written for specific therapeutic purposes that had proved effective. At the end, Maria Schüppel gave us a fascinating survey of the development of music through the ages, with characteristic samples of music of the different cultural epochs on the respective instruments. The participants of this conference are now looking forward to a further conference to take place in Camphill Glencraig in Northern Ireland in July.

Therapy with Music and Coloured Shadows

Excerpts from Karl König, 'Some Aspects on the Treatment of Cerebral Palsy', published in *Spastics Quarterly*, Christmas 1954[1]

I

It is with diffidence and hesitation that I write an article about my work with children with cerebral palsy, because I know the difficulties of conveying to the reader the basic ideas that have helped me find new ways to approach the treatment and general care of such children. On the other hand some of the results we have achieved are rather striking and it would therefore be unjustified if our methods were not made known to the general public interested in the special field of cerebral palsy ...

II

To begin with, we did not ask what we could do in order to help these children to regain their freedom of movement. Our main question was, what kind of surroundings do these children need to help ease the stress and strain under which they usually live? It was obvious that every one of them was in no way adjusted to his or her environment and our first concern was to create appropriate living conditions.

179

To this end we studied as intimately as possible the reactive behaviour of these children and soon discovered that their sense perception was grossly disturbed ...

From my own observations I sometimes wonder whether the deep disturbance within the realm of sense perception is not of at least the same importance as the disorder in muscular co-ordination. I am of the opinion that both disabilities are basically connected and are due to a common cause. Much too little attention has so far been paid to the severe derangement in the sensory sphere of the palsied patient.

III

Another very marked feature of children with athetoid cerebral palsy is their instability in the emotional sphere. Our observations reveal not only that the emotional instability is a common feature among such children, but also that special patterns of emotional and temperamental reactions are closely bound up with the different types of cerebral palsy.

Children with spastic cerebral palsy have a different emotional make-up from athetoid children, and the latter is again unlike those with more rigid types of cerebral palsy. Each one of these three types has typical emotional reactions and it is important to outline them in their fundamental characteristics.

The most obvious feature of children with spastic cerebral palsy is a pronounced appearance of fear and anxiety. Fear of the dark, fear of other human beings, fear of sitting, fear of falling are constantly present. The temperament of such children often shows a tendency to be melancholic and given to self-pity and introspection.

In athetoid children the pattern of their emotional

display is quite a different one. Their emotions are as sudden, uncontrolled and jerking as their movements. They are given to sudden outbreaks of weeping without any apparent reason and this can equally well change to sudden bursts of laughter. It is as difficult for athetoid children to stop weeping as it is for them to stop laughing, and sometimes only after a considerably period of time are they able to regain their emotional balance. They show in this display an emotional level that otherwise is only observed in early infancy. Their temperament is more sanguine and, of all types of cerebral palsy, they have the greatest difficulty in concentrating.

The rigid type is again different. The accent in the children's emotional condition is on the slow side. There are no sudden outbreaks of joy or sadness. Their feelings slowly arise and remain for a long while on the level they have reached. It is sometimes as if a thick layer lies between the children and their surroundings. They need prolonged and intense effort to find their real personalities. Their temperament can be described as phlegmatic and the slow response of children with this type of cerebral palsy to education and training is due to this feature.

All of this, however, can show how important it is to include the emotional structure of each single patient into the diagnostic approach of cerebral palsy.

Children with ataxia form a very complex group which, to my mind, should not be included in the realm of cerebral palsy. I will therefore not deal with this type in the present article.

IV

First of all the special palsied condition of the child should be taken into consideration. It is in this field that most of the research work during the last decades has been made, and in just this sphere that a great deal of remedial approach was attempted ...

Our conceptions of the interaction between muscle and nerve, our old views on the physiology of the brain, the cortical as well as the subcortical areas, are gradually breaking down and giving way to entirely new ideas that, until now, have been classified as pure nonsense ...

What we must learn to see is the following fundamental concept: every nerve in normal conditions acts as an afferent fibre. For example, in ordinary, voluntary movement the 'motor' nerve is an afferent nerve: it conducts the impulse from the muscle via the spinal cord to the 'motor' area of the cortex, thus giving the possibility of experiencing the position of the respective part or totality of the limb in movement. As soon as damage occurs to the cortex or the subcortical grey matter (subcortical or thalamic nuclei), the distorted part fires its impulses in an efferent way into the muscles and thereby gives rise to the condition of spasticity, rigidity or athetosis. Only in pathological conditions can nerves assume the 'motor' tendency, whereby involuntary movements occur. Therefore Dr Bates stressed the infantile and athetoid character of the movements evoked by stimulation and their obvious similarity to epileptic phenomena, because in the case of convulsive seizures the responsible cortical or subcortical area acts in an efferent way instead of an afferent one. This is the basic concept that underlies our attempts in the physiotherapy of cerebral palsy.

Thus we have tried to approach palsied children in a threefold way: first of all, to create an environment in which the threshold of hypersensitivity is gradually alleviated; second, to adjust the emotional disturbance, and third to inhibit the 'efferent' action of the cortical and subcortical areas in order to enable the children to establish their natural voluntary movements. I shall now try to describe in detail our efforts and the results that we have achieved.

V

I have already described the different patterns of unstable emotions experienced by children with cerebral palsy and will now deal with one method of treating them. I venture to state that such unstable emotions are not so much due to a disturbed psychological background but have their roots in the disorder of certain physiological processes. It was again Rudolf Steiner who drew our attention to the fact that the rhythmical process of breathing is intimately connected with our emotional life. The rise and fall of special emotional experiences is bound together with inhaling and exhaling. Again the unbiased observation of every patient with cerebral palsy discloses a disharmony of the whole breathing process. If we are able to establish equality within the sphere of breathing, then we help patients develop equanimity. Our experiences have more and more demonstrated that this harmony can be achieved if the children are regularly exposed to specifically designed sensory experiences.

To this end all our children with cerebral palsy are daily taken into a room that was specially built for this purpose. Ten to fifteen children are treated at one time. To the front of this room is a white screen, which the children face. Behind the screen, and completely hidden by it, are five big windows made of different coloured glass; we use blue, red, yellow, purple and green glass. When an object is placed in the space between the windows and the screen, its shadow falls on the screen. As the windows are coloured, the shadows appear in the form of coloured

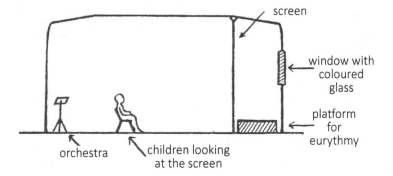

Treatment room (diagram from original article)

shadows, producing the most radiant colours. If instead of an immobile object a person performing eurythmic movements is placed between windows and screen, there appears on the latter, in constant change and beautiful splendour, ever-moving coloured shadows.

The children watch this arrangement for about twenty minutes each day. However, the coloured shadows alone would not be complete if they were not accompanied by music; therefore we have a small orchestra, consisting of two lyres and a harpsichord, and a few voices. The music and choir accompany the display of the moving coloured shadows and in this way a very soothing effect is achieved on all who attend this performance. The restless limbs become quiet, the children start to yawn and relax, and the irregular breathing in each one of them attains a regular rhythm. It is a common observation that within about ten minutes the cold hands and feet become much warmer as the blood flow is increased.

After this treatment has ended each child is put to rest in their bed or chair for a time and afterwards joins again in the daily routine.

From my personal observation and those of my colleagues I am convinced that the prolonged use of this special treatment has shown very good results. It brings about a great amount of relaxation within a group of children, and its value lies not in its form of group therapy but in alleviating the emotional stress under which the children are continuously suffering.

VI

Finally we have to turn to the treatment of the hypersensitivity of the palsied patient. Here we encounter symptoms common to all that need great care and attention ...

There is nothing more detrimental than speed and hurry, restlessness and overtaxing. The sedate speed of an old rural community is just the right measure for the life of a group of children with cerebral palsy. If this is generally observed, then within a year or two the children are gradually adjusted to bear up with our more modern ways of daily existence. But to begin with they have to be set at peace and only later, after they have gained a certain amount of emotional balance, of inner certainty and a more normal defence reaction to outer stimuli, can they be exposed to stronger experiences.

From these deliberations it will be seen that we try an all-round education of the palsied children in our care. I have only been able to mention the main points of our work ...

I nevertheless hope that this short account will give a first insight into our endeavours, which conform to the task of all who have devoted their lives to the cause of cerebral palsy, which is to give as much help as possible to those of our brethren who are in most dire need of this help.

Letters

Correspondence Between Hildebrand Richard Teirich and Karl König

Katarina Seeherr

This correspondence between Hildebrand Richard Teirich and Karl König between 1957 and 1960 describes the coming about of König's article 'Music Therapy in Curative Education' for Teirich's book *Musik in der Medizin* [Music in Medicine].[1]

The physicians Ita Wegman, Hilma Walther, Julia Bort, Hellmuth Klimm, Gisbert Husemann, Gotthard Starke, Karl König, and the musicians Edmund Pracht, Julius Knierim and Susanne Müller-Wiedemann, were all interested in applying Rudolf Steiner's indications on music for therapeutic purposes. The lecture cycle *The Inner Nature of Music and the Experience of Tone* was studied especially for this reason.

After a visit to Arlesheim in 1957, Teirich tried to get in touch with anthroposophists there, but initially received no reply. Presumably he would have turned to Julia Bort or Hilma Walther, as both had published articles about music in curative education already in 1927.[2] In the end, Teirich turned to Edmund Pracht, a friend of König's who was working in Arlesheim as a co-worker in the Further Education Courses in Medicine, Curative Education and

Music. This correspondence begins with Pracht's reply of July 8, 1957, to Teirich's letter asking if he would like to contribute to the publication of the prospective book. Pracht states:

> I have come to the conclusion, based on my experiences
> in working with physicians and, what is for me most
> important, with curative educators, that one should
> strictly distinguish between what according to their
> expertise lies within the realm of the physician on the
> one hand and that of the musician on the other. I do
> not mean this in the sense of rank, but in the sense of
> an inherent responsibility according to the nature of
> the matter in hand. Music therapy will have to prove its
> intrinsic value as an element within the overall medical
> treatment. The exact assessment of this could only be
> done by someone with a medical training who should
> be capable of being responsible for and representing the
> statements they make [in public].

Pracht considered the description of practical experiences, which, according to the above, were important to Teirich, to lie within the remit of the physician. He saw the musician's task as a different one, however, namely:

> ... to prepare the musical 'subject-matter' (the
> elements of music and the instrument), materially
> and conceptually, in such a way that possibilities for
> the practical use of music in medicine become visible
> to therapists, so that as physician, nurse and curative
> educator, independently from their connection to music,
> they will be able to understand and use it from the point
> of view of the relationship between the image of the
> human being and the range of musical phenomena.[3]

Pracht wanted a larger group of people to become acquainted with the indications given by Steiner and this could only be done by someone who was musically literate. Physicians do not usually have any musical training, although in this particular instance Pracht knew of one who did. He gave Teirich König's address and apologised for his delay in replying. Four days later, on July 12, 1957, Teirich wrote to König:

> Dear Dr König,
> You will probably not remember me – in 1938 I was often with you in Vienna. Yet it might be more likely that you remember my ex-wife (Furtwängler). I often think of you, and every now and then I hear about you from patients, but this was not the reason for contacting you.
> A contract has been drawn up between Fischer Press in Stuttgart, formerly in Jena, which states that I should take on the publication of a book with the title 'Musik in der Medizin'.
> About sixteen authors will be contributing to this scientific work. During my short stay in Arlesheim I became aware of the efforts in music therapy being made, and for this reason I would very much welcome a contribution from the anthroposophical side.

Teirich mentioned that his efforts to find anthroposophical contributors had so far been unsuccessful and that two physicians and the 'Council in Dornach' had not replied at all. Mr Pracht, however, who understood his efforts, had referred him to König.

> Could I ask you to provide an article written by you? In the German-speaking world there is, at this time, no book available that is directed to the physician and I do think this is needed. In the first lines one's own

practical experiences should be discussed in a form that is scientific, yet understandable, allowing also those interested in musicology to be part of the readership.

A deadline of October 10 was given for the article, and a fee of 100–150 deutschmarks was offered. An edition of 2,500 copies was being planned. Teirich asked König to reply soon so that he would be able to finalise the list of contributors.

It is interesting that Teirich already knew Karl König from his time in Vienna where he visited him often before he emigrated. Teirich also heard about König via the latter's patients, although by then König had been living in Scotland for almost twenty years.

Nearly two weeks later, on July 30, 1957, Karl König replied. He thanked Teirich for his letter and said that he remembered him very clearly. He also thanked him for advice on the article, which he planned to write it in the holidays. However, König did not want the term 'anthroposophy' to appear in the title or anywhere else because 'I do not want to be stamped as being part of a sect.' The reason for this may be found in König's problematic relationship with 'the anthroposophists' in Dornach.[4]

In August 1957 Teirich informed all the contributors that the book would be published in Spring 1958. He reminded them that it should be expected that musicologists will be among the readers and that they should 'take this into account in the way you write the article.'

A handwritten note by König mentioned that his article, along with the biographical note that Teirich had requested from all contributors, was sent by registered post on October 3, one week before the article's deadline.

In a note on October 11 to all contributors, Teirich confirmed the he had received König's work, and in a short personal remark to König he said, 'By just glancing through your article I can already see that you have put a lot of work into it.'

On November 11, Teirich wrote to König, telling him that he had finished reading the last of the manuscripts, including König's article:

> I feel the urge to express my special gratitude to you. Your work has a significantly scientific format, contains material that is fundamentally new to non-anthroposophists, and will appeal to very many readers.

Teirich very much wanted to speak to König about some urgent questions and asked when he would again be in Germany. He also complimented König on his German, which had not suffered at all despite his long stay abroad. For the other articles Teirich would have to appoint a German language specialist to 'translate' the German writings into German.

On September 1, 1958, Teirich wrote to the contributors informing them that *Musik in der Medizin* had gone to print.

On November 8, Teirich wrote to König asking if he had received his complimentary copies of the book yet. But the real reason for the letter was to ask König for advice in relation to a sixteen-year-old patient whom Teirich very much wanted to see admitted to one of König's homes.

König replied on November 14, apologising that he was unable to admit the patient in question but that he could recommend him to another pedagogue. On the publication of the book he writes:

> In the meantime, my complimentary copy of *Musik in der Medizin* has arrived and looks excellent to me. Its layout and print are immaculate, and I am incredibly grateful that I could be one of the contributors to this important

work. I would like to thank you very much for this and congratulate you on the publication.

König asked to be informed about the response to the book in the professional press, and in reply to Teirich's question concerning when he would next be Germany, he wrote that it would probably be soon after Easter the following year. König then asked whether Teirich would be able to organise a lecture at his college in Freiburg so that he could speak about Camphill.[5]

On January 29, 1959, Teirich wrote to König to ask if he would give a 45-minute lecture to 400–500 physicians at a 'Day for Music Therapy', which he was going to organise in Velden am Wörthersee. About the book he writes:

> The music book is doing surprisingly well – are people in England also speaking about it? From Palestine alone five copies have been ordered, as well as already some from the USA – only via word of mouth, as order forms have not been sent out yet.

On February 10, 1959, König replied to Teirich apologising that he was unable to give the lecture in Velden due to prior commitments, but that he would still be able to give the lecture in Freiburg: 'This would enable us to see each other again and I am looking forward to this very much.'

On February 20, König replied to another letter from Teirich (not available), in which he said that he would be speaking to the Physicians' Society in Innsbruck on May 6 and would like to meet up with Teirich on May 7 – most likely with his colleague Dr Hans Heinrich Engel and with Alix Roth who accompanied König on his journeys. Two planned lectures about curative education in Camphill would then be given to any interested physicians and students the following day.

Teirich replied to König on March 18 that he would send out invitations to the lectures in Freiburg, and he asked to be mentioned to the physicians at Innsbruck:

> I would be much obliged to you if you could mention my name in Innsbruck. Innsbruck was my first leading position in 1947 and I did not have much success with my proposals for reform ... The book is doing quite well. So far, we have had six reviews, mostly positive, apart from one from a colleague from Vienna who wrote that he did not see any therapeutic possibility in music.

The correspondence comes to an end with a circular by Teirich to all contributors to the book in December 1960:

> It has now been two years since the publication of *Musik in der Medizin* and I would like to make use of this occasion to let you know that, according to the publisher, the success of the work is very satisfactory for a scientific book. So far, about seventy reviews have appeared, almost all positive and many even enthusiastic. I must admit that I had not at all expected this. There are a few critical opinions, and the individual articles are discussed partly in a surprisingly knowledgeable and very exhaustive way. Of the total number of reviews four are guarded. Only one 'review', from Mr Pontvik, was 'crushing', but, as it was not at all based on facts, it was corrected by the journal itself.

In this circular Teirich also reported on the first Conference on Music Therapy held in September 1959 in Velden am Wörthersee, and on the new music therapy training in Vienna. In conclusion he introduced the international music journal *Heilkunst* [The Art of

Healing] which had a positive reception and was discussed extensively several times:

> In any case, the journal in its definitive version by far exceeded a report about a conference and constitutes an important complement to the book *Musik in der Medizin*. Further publications will follow and I hope that I may again approach you if need be.

With the help of the correspondence between Teirich and König it is possible to see behind the scenes and to accompany the process of the coming about of *Musik in der Medizin*. Teirich and König renewed their acquaintance from their Vienna days and set up a meeting in Freiburg. Unfortunately, nothing could be found out about the urgent questions that Teirich wished to discuss with König.

Correspondence Between Hermann Pfrogner and Karl König

Katarina Seeherr

In the introduction to his autobiography, *Leben und Werk* [Life and Work], after mentioning the results of his musicological research, Hermann Pfrogner writes: 'And, finally, I have attempted to help to bring about the spiritual-scientific foundation of a future music therapy'.[1]

What follows is a short overview of Pfrogner's life and his path towards music therapy, including his meeting with Karl König, which brought about a new impulse for anthroposophical music therapy. This was documented in Hans Heinrich Engel's *Musical Anthropology* and in the correspondence between Pfrogner and Engel.[2] In Pfrogner, König encountered a person who had found the aspect of life-forces in music in his own specific way and who, as a scientist, was also able to record them. König's life-long striving for an understanding of the living, which might well have begun with his lecture at the Embryological Institute in Vienna in 1925, culminated in the area of music through this encounter.

Hermann Pfrogner went to school in Innsbruck. He studied counterpoint and composition in Vienna at the state music academy while simultaneously studying law at the university. He concluded his studies in 1934. After the war he also studied musicology in Vienna. During the Second World War, while he was a radio operator in the Russia campaign, a new theme suddenly became important to him:

> Through the theory of harmony I became acquainted
> with keynote, dominant and sub-dominant as static
> concepts, and now the thought occurred to me that it
> is really a play of forces and that one has to attempt to
> grasp the two forces of dominant and subdominant in a
> dynamic way and see the keynote as the balance between
> the two.[3]

After having worked together with Johann Nepomuk David[4] for a time in Stuttgart, Pfrogner went on a lecture tour. He wrote the following about his lectures at a conference in Bayreuth in 1939, which he gave on the theme of 'Youth and Music':

> It is important to note that in Bayreuth I addressed for
> the first time the important overcoming of space and
> time within enharmonics.

After the lecture, the German composer Fritz Büchtger[5] spoke to him and advised him to get in touch with Anny von Lange, which Pfrogner did in 1950. He writes about her:

> This brilliant woman – for this is what she was –
> introduced me to anthroposophy systematically, step by
> step, in a manner that was very inspiring.

Anny von Lange's life's work, however, was devoted to Goethean research into music. She invited Pfrogner to give a lecture at a summer conference organised by her in Bad Liebenzell. Pfrogner took up this challenge every year. From 1953 onwards these conferences took place in a college in Holland called Land en Bosch. In 1956 Anny von Lange fell ill and Pfrogner had to lead the conference at short notice. Pfrogner took this initiative further with help of musicians Otto Crusius, Wilhelm Dörfler and Fritz Büchtger:

> In March 1962 I had one of the most decisive
> experiences of my life. In 1961 I had been asked by the
> Dutch friends to speak about the etheric nature of the
> intervals. In relation to this I found in Rudolf Steiner's
> lecture cycle *Man in the Light of Occultism, Theosophy and
> Philosophy* in the ninth lecture the 'seven members of
> the inner human being in movement', the 'seven inner
> movements, which are: the movement of uprightness,
> the thinking movement, the speech movement,
> the blood movement, the breathing movement,
> the glandular movement and the movement of
> reproduction.'[6] The sequence in the way they were given
> looks at the origin of movement. Already when only
> reading these words, the corresponding diatonic intervals
> came to me, and when looking at the origin of the
> intervals I immediately saw before me musical examples
> from the compositions of certain composers. I presented
> these ideas at the Summer Conference in Land en Bosch
> in 1962 and elicited great interest from the members of
> the Camphill movement who were attending. They were
> the excellent singer Veronika Bay, her sister Ursula and
> her husband Rudolf Geraets, who lived near Utrecht
> in Christophorus.[7] They immediately informed the
> founder of the movement, Dr Karl König, a brilliant
> medical doctor, of what they had heard. He then visited
> me in the autumn in Stuttgart, where I played to him

the intervals of the 'seven inner movements' on the piano. His delighted comment was: 'Finally a musician!' He appeared to be extremely moved by the intervals demonstrated to him, which was the reason why the friends at Christophorus invited me to the next clinic[8] to be held at their place.[9]

At Easter 1963, Pfrogner took part in the workshop and in the college meeting at Christophorus. After intensive phenomenological studies, which also included eurythmy, Hans Heinrich Engel and the music therapists were able to incorporate his ideas about the inner movements of the human being into music therapy treatments. Then, in the autumn of 1963, Pfrogner visited König in the residential special school Brachenreuthe where:

> Dr König challenged me to also occupy myself with the 'Seven Life Processes'. I then had a look at Rudolf Steiner's lecture cycle *The Riddle of Humanity* and for the first time I read the seventh lecture on breathing, warming, nourishing, secreting, maintaining, growing and reproducing. From my point of view I was from the first moment onwards convinced that only the diatonic intervals could correspond to these life-processes, but which ones?[10]

After his intensive work with the life processes, what became known as the 'Life Curve' came about. This is a tonal sequence that encompasses all the life processes and which has become an integral part of contemporary music therapy. During Easter, 1964, Pfrogner presented his findings in relation to the life processes and the intervals to Engel and König; on Ascension Day he familiarised them with the 'life-force-curve' he had developed. Both doctors called it a breakthrough.[11] König commented on

Pfrogner's findings in a way that showed how pleased he was:

I am extremely pleased that the seven life processes have found a music-therapeutic foundation, because I believe that we should look for the roots of our efforts there.[12]

Pfrogner considered himself to be a musicologist, not a music therapist. For this reason it was important to him that the results of his research were observed and further researched in a phenomenological way by medical doctors, eurythmists and music therapists. In the 'friends of Christophorus', and with Hans Heinrich Engel and Karl König as medical doctors, Pfrogner had found the right people at the right time in the right place, making it possible for something fruitful to come about.

The correspondence between Pfrogner and König and the friends in Christophorus gives a picture of the collaboration between Pfrogner and König. König's death and Pfrogner's illness at the time brought this correspondence to an end, but the theme was researched further and the impulse lived on in Camphill communities in the Netherlands, Northern Ireland, Scotland and Switzerland, as well as in Berlin in the Center for Music Therapy (Musiktherapeutische Arbeitsstätte), the first anthroposophical school for music therapists founded by Maria Schüppel in 1963. One can read more on this in the work by Engel and by Iris Jacobeit mentioned above.

The following correspondence with Hermann Pfrogner describes how Dr König was involved in the development of music therapy and how his ideas were taken up.

From Hermann Pfrogner's letter to Veronika Bay, February 4, 1963[13]

Dear Miss Bay,

A week ago I received a letter from Dr König in which he gave me the exact dates of his visit to Germany ... So far, everyone whom I have talked to about the relationship between the inner movements and the musical intervals in the way I presented it to you over the summer has been spontaneously convinced about it. This fills me with great joy. Now I would still like to speak to Dr König about it before I come, and I hope that we will be able to thrash out the various possibilities for the practical applications in our work together. These things can definitely be applied to Curative Eurythmy, too. It would be lovely if we could also make progress in this area and if Miss Reeskamp or another eurythmist could take part.

Hermann Pfrogner's letter to the Friends in Glencraig[14] and Christophorus, May 20, 1963

My dear Friends in Glencraig and Christophorus,

It is time for me to tell you about a conversation I was able to have with Dr König just a week ago in Brachenreuthe Residential School near Überlingen/Bodensee. Already before my journey to the Netherlands I was able to present to Dr König the correspondences that had come to me between the diatonic intervals and the inner movements [that] Rudolf Steiner spoke about, and he assured me then that he fully agreed with me. I was even more pleased to be able to tell him about the great results of our gathering at Easter. I also have certain questions which burden me and which I wanted to put before him, such as for instance, how far it is allowed to discuss things that we have learned in writing and not just by word of mouth. Dr König allayed my misgivings as he is of the opinion that we should not be too worried in this respect, and in the light of this I am now sending you the pages included in this letter.

Since we parted from each other I have been working intensively on the intervals and the texts, and I hope that I am now able to send you the final versions. I would very much like to show these versions to Dr König as well and to get his opinion. In relation to this, Dr König said that in the case of the 'thinking' movement (microcosmically speaking) one could say that one can feel that it is lit up or darkened 'through me', and that this could not be said about the 'blood' movement. I initially crossed out these words in my text. Dr König was unwilling to comment on the fact that Dr Engel had put so much emphasis on the 'through me', especially in the case of the blood movement. As you can see, I have nevertheless re-inserted these words into the text and will also explain this to Dr König to whom I had sent the first version of the text. Apart from through the musical experience of the interval, I would definitely be unable to say that I can feel whether or not the blood movement becomes lighter or darker 'through me'. Yet this is different when I experience the blood movement through music. The significance of music for certain experiences is that in music things and experiences can appear to people that normally cannot be experienced at all. In the minor third I experienced this lightening or darkening 'through me' all the time so strongly that I was unable to decide whether to remove these words in relation to the experience of the musical interval.

In connection with the 'breathing' movement, König made the additional remark that hyperventilation could mean a darkening process to our consciousness as in certain circumstances it could lead to fainting. From this point of view, each inhalation would also be a slight process of falling asleep. In this sense, spring is the beginning of the earth's sleep. This was never meant to be an additional remark to what Dr Engel presented in relation to inhalation and exhalation. As for the 'glandular' movement, Dr König thought that the expression 'to gland' was linguistically rather ugly. Therefore I decided in my manuscript to change it into the verb 'to dew', which might be the most meaningful in relation to the noun 'dew' for this movement from a macrocosmic-microcosmic viewpoint.

What Dr König said about the function of the mirrored forms of the archetypes of the breathing movement and the movement of reproducing was very interesting, but I have been unable to find any notes on this from Christophorus. In relation to the mirrored interval sequence of the breathing movement – the ascending-descending minor sixth and the descending-ascending major third – Dr König said that it seemed to him like this had something to do with 'flying' (minor sixth, up–down) and 'landing' (major third, down–up). The flying bird releases warmth, for instance, and is as if being taken hold of by the winged forces of the universe. In relation to the mirrored interval sequence of the movement of reproducing – the diminished fifth ascending–descending, the augmented fourth, descending–ascending – Dr König said that this is connected with 'knowing' (diminished fifth up–down), and 'hearing' (augmented fourth down–up).

Dr König expressed his agreement with the qualifications 'active' and passive', which I had recently added to the individual archetypes. It was because of these additional qualifications of 'active' and passive' that I was able to explore the experience of the different intervals further. In this way a threefold grouping appears. In experiencing the intervals of the movements of thinking, blood and glands, activity is needed in order to form a relationship to the macrocosm. The movements of speech, breathing and reproducing, on the other hand, depend on the gods first becoming active and imparting these forms of movement to us as divine gifts. Dr König fully agreed with this and added the wonderful remark that the active impulse for the thinking movement is given by the 'ego-self', the one to the blood movement by the 'ego-form within me' and the one to the glandular movement by the 'angel in me'.

Based on the newly added qualifications 'active' and 'passive' it also occurred to me that the archetypes in hearing, singing and eurythmy can be divided in the following way:

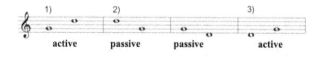

Thus, a three-folding arises, as you can see. In this way it can be experienced even more clearly how the fifth, 'by the grace of the octave' as I put it in Christophorus, presents us with the fourth, etc. The rhythm between 'activity' and 'passivity', moreover, presents us with totally new experiences. Instead of 'active', one could also say 'male' and instead of 'passive', 'female'. Archetypically they can be compared to the Chinese 'yang' and 'yin'. The interplay between male and female is thus expressed vividly. It is possible to follow this up with the individual intervals as forms of movement, and with each interval it will lead to special discoveries that I do not want to go into any further here as most of it is self-evident.

Dr König appeared to be quite moved by the description of the Saturday afternoon and evening, where we occupied ourselves for the first time with the blood movement, then experienced the eve of Emmaus after which I was able to tell you a bit about the interval F–F# and the etherisation. As Dr König has no problem with this, I am now able to tell you that it seems to me that with the following interval sequence, Dr Engel exactly pointed to what Rudolf Steiner described about 'the experience of major' and 'the experience of minor' in relation to the Christ experience.[15]

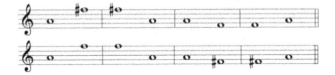

Interestingly, both Christoph Andreas [Lindenberg] and I were under the impression that here the major third is experienced as if it is minor and the minor third as if it is major. It seems to me that these things are pointing to a first hint of something unfathomable. For this we must be especially grateful to Dr Engel but also to Miss Reeskamp (to her, especially, in relation to the tritone and the dangers surrounding it; I will never forget this moment!)

Dr König also seemed very impressed with what I had pointed to in relation to the sequence at the end of the Emmaus-evening. He wants to give special attention to this interval sequence. Dr König attributed a special significance to the constellation of this Saturday, because, he said, 'such things always occur when the moon is in Pisces'. In his conclusion Dr König called our Easter conference shattering and he stated that he very much wants to take part in next year's conference in Christophorus as well.

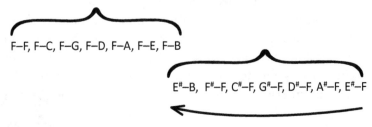

F–F, F–C, F–G, F–D, F–A, F–E, F–B

E#–B, F#–F, C#–F, G#–F, D#–F, A#–F, E#–F

Dr König had told me already before Easter in Stuttgart that he considered the connection of the seven diatonic intervals with the seven inner movements to be an 'ingenious, new starting point for music therapy'. This impression became even stronger for him after the description of our Easter conference. This is where we stand at this moment. We have now reached the first stage that has given a new starting point from the music itself. That which I as a musician was able to do by connecting the intervals with the movements has led to a certain outcome that forms an acceptable basis. Now the second stage begins and it is the turn of the physicians. Dr König said that he wanted to meet with Dr Engel, Chr. Andr. Lindenberg et al in order to discuss a concrete, therapeutic evaluation from a medical point of view. Dr König will be passing through Munich as part of a lecture tour in the autumn. He would then like to meet up with me again over here. And, as I mentioned earlier, he also wants to take part in our conference in Christophorus the following spring. He thought that we could extend the number of participants to up to thirty. It will probably be quite a gradual process before we need to make this number our limit.

I also had the opportunity to get to know the matron of Brachenreuthe and three young co-workers who are specially occupied with music over there. Things promise to be very fruitful there. Last Monday afternoon I was able to speak with Dr König for a total of five hours, and on Tuesday lunchtime for another one-and-a-half hours. Dr König was so kind as to collect me from the station and take me to my hotel and the next day again to the train. When saying goodbye he said that 'these were very memorable 25 hours', the total time I had spent here – from my side I can only confirm this with gratitude.

I have made four copies of the enclosed pages.[16] Dr König will receive the original. There is one copy for the

Friends in Glencraig and Christophorus. I would like to ask Mrs Slotemaker and Mrs Reeskamp to make copies themselves, as my typewriter is unable to make so many copies. I am still with you all in thought,

   With kind regards,
   Yours,
   Hermann Pfrogner

Letter to Karl König, February 2, 1964

My very dear Dr König,
   You will have heard from Ms Herbig about the working conference held at the beginning of the year in Munich where, unexpectedly, a task was set by the spiritual world to take up a confrontation with evil 'that would fall in with the fruitful spiritual forces of human development in order to cooperate towards the good'. These insights, which were imparted to me here by the grace of the spiritual world, are related to the possible resolution of the problem which you yourself pointed out to me in Brachenreuthe after I had heard from our Dutch friends how much this subject had occupied you – namely, how to approach the seven life processes through music therapy: breathing-consuming, warming-combusting, nourishing-sedimentation, etc.

   If the problem was solved – and I believe and hope it was – then a great step forward was made over the threshold of music therapy after the door to this had first been nudged open by the insight into the correspondence between the 'seven-fold division of the inner, mobile human being', and the sevenfold diatonic intervals in the way they have come about.

   Because of the intensity, well known to you, with which I have put my energies into the founding of a music therapy based on the archetypal elements of music, you will understand when I tell you: I live every day only for the moment after Easter in Christophorus (the Dutch friends will still tell me the exact starting date of the conference) in which I will be able to let you know what we learned and worked on in Munich. And one other thing: please do not study my written pages, which Ms Herbig brought you; they are very incomplete and only present a one-sided picture full of gaps! Please wait for the direct meeting with the phenomena!

In heartfelt expectation of seeing each other again,

Yours,

Hermann Pfrogner

Letter from Karl König, February 19, 1964

My very dear Dr Pfrogner!

The time after Christmas was so endlessly full with lectures, courses, meetings and not least with preparation for our move to Germany, that it has not been possible to study what you sent me by hand of Ms Herbig. Please understand this and do not consider it to be a lack of interest.

I am extremely pleased that the seven life processes have found a music-therapeutic foundation, because I believe that we should look for the roots of our efforts there. I will take all your notes with me and will then write again from Brachenreuthe. Our meeting after Easter in Christophorus, however, will be most important. I am very much looking forward to it and will try and find some time for the necessary preparation.

With many good wishes and heartfelt greetings,

as always yours,

Karl König

Letter from Hermann Pfrogner, February 23, 1964

My very dear Dr König!

This letter, which I am directing to you in the name of Christophorus – where I am also at present – is about the forthcoming Easter gathering. When I reported to you in Brachenreuthe on the outcomes of the last Easter meeting you recommended to me, on the basis of these outcomes, that I occupy myself with the seven life impulses and their degeneration. After the beginning of the working week in Munich with Ms Reeskamp, during the second half of the Holy Nights the spiritual world gave me a completely unexpected nudge to translate your challenge into deeds. Mrs Herbig brought you a first draft of the musical results and in my subsequent letter I asked you to put this draft aside for the time being and to wait for the meeting with the phenomena in Christophorus.

Due to the inner necessity that appeared out of the results from Munich, Christophorus, including Dr Engel, out of a freely made decision and hoping that you would understand, changed the theme of the forthcoming Easter gathering. The achievements from Munich need the approval of professional physicians. This approval will be the exclusive theme of the forthcoming conference. In this way the circle will be organically completed which began with the challenge given to me in Brachenreuthe. We would kindly ask you all to agree with this change of theme.

The fact that we are trying here to gain a first approval by the physicians and a way to express very intimate musical phenomena that arise from a confrontation with the influences of the counter forces, it seems advisable to limit the number of participants as much as possible. Our proposal is that, apart from the present co-workers from Christophorus, only you and Miss Roth, Dr Engel and his wife, and Christoph Andreas Lindenberg as a representative from Camphill and myself would take part. It is also the case that Christophorus feels that they are at present unable to host a larger number of participants, because the number of children that will stay on over Easter will be larger than it was last year.

In the hope that I will also have your understanding on this point, and looking forward to our forthcoming reunion in Christophorus, I am sending you heartfelt greetings in the name of all the friends.

Yours,

Dr Hermann Pfrogner

Letter from Hermann Pfrogner, November 22, 1964

My very dear Dr König!

Today, as promised, I will give you a short description of what I understand by diatonic, chromatic and enharmonic.

We will only be able to get closer to these musical facts if we call on the inherent inner-hearing experience of our musicality, the inner orientation of hearing of our inherent musicality. Just as we have a disposition for orientation in order to find our way in the world, so do we also have a disposition for an inner musical-hearing orientation that helps us find our way in the musical world. The word 'disposition' means that we are not born with this inner musical hearing orientation 'ripe and ready', but that it first has to be developed, just as we also otherwise have to find the right way in the world.

The hearing orientation formed with the help of the above disposition becomes active step by step in different, staggered layers, which, so to speak, have been arranged one behind the other.

The primary layer of our musical-hearing orientation that comes first into action corresponds to the diatonic.

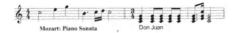

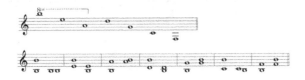

By 'diatonic' I do not primarily mean the various keys or major or minor, but the seven types of intervals that come about in pairs if you put together seven tones that occur within an octave, with fifths (or fourths) between each one.

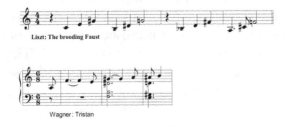

When coming across a piece of music, we will always try to find our way into it diatonically at first. No one would get the idea to presume that, for instance in our Mozart example, there would be the interval of C–F♭ instead of C–E.

It would be possible, however, that we come across some musical situations where this layer of the diatonic hearing orientation that comes to mind first is not enough:

Here we can only find the right way if the next layer in our inner-hearing orientation, corresponding to chromatics, comes into action. It may be the case that in a person the first layer of hearing orientation is functioning, but not the second that lies behind it. Such a person will understand our Mozart examples, but not the Liszt or the Wagner ones.

In another example, someone for whom the first layer of the hearing orientation does not function – who therefore does not really find their way into our Mozart examples – will not under any circumstances be able to find their way into the Liszt and Wagner examples.

Chromatics can manifest in two ways:

1. By raising or lowering the tone of an interval, so that again only a diatonic interval comes about:

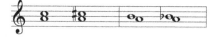

2. By raising or lowering the tone of an interval, so that an augmented or diminished (and with it a chromatic) interval comes about:

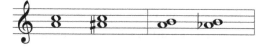

In the latter case the musical context makes it inevitable that either an $A^\#$ or an $A^\flat$ occurs. If you play the latter interval on the piano, the first layer of our hearing orientation will immediately present itself and register:

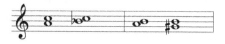

In no way should chromatics be understood to be the twelve keys of the piano in the sense of the so-called 'chromatic scale'. This is a totally false concept which, unfortunately, has come into the public domain because of the sloppiness of musical theory.

In chromatics each tonal value can be raised or lowered once or twice over:

$$\longleftrightarrow$$

$$C^{bb} - C^b - C - C^\# - C*$$
$$D^{bb} - D^b - D - D^\# - D*$$
$$E^{bb} - E^b - E - E^\# - E*$$
$$F^{bb} - F^b - F - F^\# - F*$$
$$G^{bb} - G^b - G - G^\# - G*$$
$$A^{bb} - A^b - A - A^\# - A*$$
$$B^{bb} - B^b - B - B^\# - B*$$

Our usual diatonic-chromatic tonal provision, as it has come about out of the chromatic differentiation of the seven diatonic keynotes, therefore consists of 35 tonal values (5×7).

There are, however, other musical relationships that we can encounter in the course of a musical piece, in which neither the first, the 'diatonic' layer, nor the second, the 'chromatic' layer, of our inner hearing orientation suffice.

In our orientation we can really only grasp this if, apart from the two afore-mentioned so-called layers of our inner hearing orientation, an additional layer lying behind the other ones comes into action that corresponds to enharmonics.

Enharmonics can occur in two forms:

1. As a transformation of one tonal value into another one – as if on the flip side of the page – where a $G^\#$ changes into a A^b. Here we speak of an enharmonic modulation (from A-minor to C-minor.)

2. As a mutual interpenetration of two tonal values as in the following example:

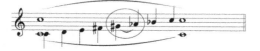

This time there is no modulation, no transition from one tonality into another, no change-over from $G^{\#}$ to $A^{\flat}$. The tone C that is being sustained as a whole note remains a diatonic basis for the whole. An interpenetration comes about here from $G^{\#}$ to $A^{\flat}$, both being present simultaneously. In such a case I am speaking about enharmonic integration.

In both cases where enharmonics occur, it is striking that our notation system is not equipped to provide a realistic picture. Our notation system can depict diatonic and chromatic relationships flawlessly, but it can only express a $G^{\#}$ and an $A^{\flat}$ if they are beside each other, not the transformation from $G^{\#}$ into $A^{\flat}$ (and vice versa) or the interpenetration of $G^{\#}$ and $A^{\flat}$.

In order to fully understand enharmonics the deepest, most hidden layer of our inner-hearing orientation is called upon, namely the disposition of our musicality to summarise the manifold diatonic-chromatic tonal variety from $F^{\flat}$ to $B^{\#}$ into twelve tonal centres. I mean here by 'tonal centre' the qualitative correlate, inherent in our musicality, to the qualitative pitch as represented in the frequencies of the twelve keynotes of the piano.

In the case of enharmonics, the actual piano key has three different meanings:

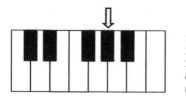

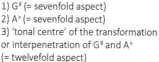

1) $G^{\#}$ (= sevenfold aspect)
2) $A^{\flat}$ (= sevenfold aspect)
3) 'tonal centre' of the transformation or interpenetration of $G^{\#}$ and $A^{\flat}$ (= twelvefold aspect)

The open and, as such, continually differentiating manifoldness of the now commonly known 35 diatonic-chromatic tonal values from F$^\flat$ to B$^\sharp$ is only rounded off into a wholeness by the cooperation of the sevenfold and the twelvefold aspects.

So much for diatonics, chromatics and enharmonics. What here takes place musically has been musical reality ever since Wagner and Debussy, but is by far not yet known. On the contrary, the catch phrase 'Debussy the impressionist' has managed to beautifully stop up our hearing and make it superficial.

Otherwise, however, I am of the opinion that in the case of the relationship of the seven diatonic intervals to the 'seven forms of movements' we are first and foremost dealing with the etheric. Here we must distinguish between two things:

1. The individual interval in the way it proceeds successively, for example:

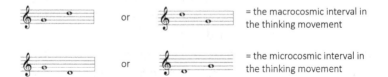

= the macrocosmic interval in the thinking movement

= the microcosmic interval in the thinking movement

2. The archetypal interval sequences that I gave at Easter, 1963, in Christophorus, of which I provided the

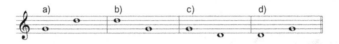

following texts at the time:

a) *I feel* how the thinking of the gods opens up to me that which works in the cosmos as the archetype of my thinking movement.

b) *I feel* how the feeling of the gods penetrates down
into me, etc.

c) *I feel* how thinking space expands within me.

d) *I feel* how I unite myself by thinking.

When feeling oneself into the above interval sequences,
astrality reigns there. And when Robert Schumann connects
the interval (d) with his 'Dreaming', the microcosmic
interval of the thinking movement is naturally interwoven
by astrality.

But when looking at them individually, we are in the
realm of the etheric with the seven diatonic intervals. How
else would it be possible, as you, Dr König, very rightly said
in Christophorus, that in the following the etheric aspects
(Adam: female ether body, Eve: male ether body) stand
before us (and it is definitely true that these are etheric
bodies).

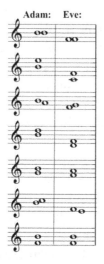

As to their origin, these aspects, however, exactly
correspond to the inner movements.

Heartfelt greetings from Hermann Pfrogner.

NB. A carbon copy of this letter is being sent to Dr
Engel so he can be in the picture at the same time.

Letter from Hermann Pfrogner, June 18, 1965

My very dear Dr König!

You would have noticed when we met again in Munich that my heart was full to bursting with what needed to be reported about St Prex.[17] Yet the evening was so much geared to the subject of the 'Village Community',[18] and it seemed to me that your strength was so much taken up by this, that it was clear from the start that any further discussions had to be postponed.

Today I will also keep it short. A foundation stone laying ceremony took place in St Prex at Whitsun. This foundation stone is a reality and has been put in the ground at St Prex. It is not by any means clear when a music therapy or art therapy institute will arise above it. This will initially depend on how the practical changeover of St Prex to the movement-work will unfold, and then also on how much Johanna Spalinger will be able to free herself for the essential tasks which she would have to fulfil in such an institute, which is not easy. Besides these things, some questions still need to be answered. Nevertheless, there is no doubt that there is a fundamental possibility for such an institute at St Prex – and only there – and that the foundation stone has been laid.

People seemed to have been deeply impressed with what I presented during the conference. This became clear to me by the many shining eyes, often filled with tears, when we said goodbye. I think I may say that every participant went home with the conviction that there will one day be a 'teachable and learnable' music therapy in existence. The fact that Dr Engel will hardly be available for St Prex any longer, from the medical point of view, is a great loss, which will not easily be filled.

This summer I will attempt to formulate in writing, greatly relying upon my lectures in St Prex, the musicological knowledge that I have gained in relation to the life processes and the inner movements. My dear Dr König, you once said that at first we all only had an inkling of an inkling of what was being given to us with this knowledge. And believe me that the experience of an inkling is, and will be, an inkling that will fill me most deeply when doing this work. With this publication a gate will be opened to possibilities for a music therapy that at present can hardly be surmised. May the sluice gates that will be opened with this make space only for water full of blessings, so the dried out, barren land may be re-enlivened. This is my innermost wish to the spiritual world.

My heartfelt greetings to you as the guardian spirit of a music therapy that is realistic, teachable and learnable.

Yours,

Dr Hermann Pfrogner

Letter from Karl König, June 21, 1965

My very dear Dr Pfrogner,

Your letter of June 18 gave me the greatest pleasure. I knew exactly why you did not speak about St Prex on Monday evening and I thank you for your kind consideration and insight.

What you wrote about your conviction that a foundation stone was laid in St Prex over which a musical or even a complete artistic therapy institute will be erected fills me with great pleasure. May it be so! I myself will attempt to devote more time to this task from now onwards and to help St Prex make progress in becoming part of the Camphill movement so that the intended tasks in relation to music therapy may be taken up as soon as possible.

I send you my best wishes for the completion of the book you are intending to write this summer.[19] It will be the husk of the seed that will be laid into the soil of St Prex. We hope that this husk will allow new seeds to germinate within it again and again so that those who enjoy them will be nourished and enthused by the new thing they will bring about.

My heartfelt gratitude to you for what you are helping to build up with such great devotion.

Very affectionately yours,

Karl König

Letter from Hermann Pfrogner to Dr Hans Heinrich Engel and the friends at Christophorus March 3, 1970

Dear Hans Heinrich, Dear Dutch Friends, Dear Johanna and Hans Spalinger,

[*Pfrogner gives an extensive report of the recent 'Schüppel conference' in the newly founded Centre for Music Therapy in Berlin. He describes this as a historic achievement.*]

There is only one comparable case to this and, as we are now approaching Easter, it goes back seven years: it was the gathering in Christophorus after Easter, 1963, when we worked on the intervals of the inner movements for the first time. And now it was again just as it was then. It was exactly the right time, there were exactly the right people and it was the right place. Seven years ago, in autumn, Dr König challenged me to occupy myself with the life processes. And these were the seven most intensive years in which we went through highs and lows, and which have now finally led to a very satisfactory and sound achievement. We know who the people were who then came together seven years ago in Christophorus. It was a strange coincidence that Miss Schüppel was then with us, as she was also in the summer of 1964 in Land en Bosch at the last conference of the group founded by

Anny von Lange. I can still see Maria Schüppel standing before me when, together with some others, I tried out the 'Life Curve' in eurythmy, which I had already shown to Dr König and Hans Heinrich on Ascension Day, 1964, when Maria Schüppel also took part. This is just an indication of the wonderful thread that is mysteriously running through everything that was achieved in relation to the present conference in Berlin.

Hermann Pfrogner

Notebooks

On the Ear and Hearing

I

Notes for a lecture given in London on November 6, 1943

I

1. The mystery of the human ear. Still we do not know
   how hearing is performed. The organ of Corti (1860)
   discovered. Many theories, but no solution.
2. This organ of Corti only to be found in mammalians.
   All the other vertebrates have no cochlea! The
   invertebrates have no such organ at all.
3. The organ of Corti is only in animals who have
   developed a kind of possibility to sound from within.

II

1. The question of the double-organ: equilibrium-hearing.
   Why is our sense of equilibrium entirely connected
   with the sense of hearing?
2. The sense of equilibrium in the animal kingdom:

   vertebrates

   invertebrates

3. The difference.

III

1. To understand the whole question we must ask: How are sounds produced? Movement!
2. Sound is the light and movement the shadow! Motion – Emotion.
3. More motion – less hearing; more hearing – less motion.

IV

1. The ear is an organ to bring movement to rest.
2. Anatomy of the ear.
3. Physiology of the ear.

V

1. Once all animals could hear. They went into movement and lost their hearing!
2. They started to sound and became listeners again.
3. Humankind acquired speech and thus became complete hearers.

II

Notes for a lecture given in London on November 7, 1943

I

1. We have tried to understand yesterday that hearing is a gift that all creatures possess.
   The lower animals are ears and we have only to understand how having ears develops from being ears more and more. A kind of all-round hearing changes then into a individualised hearing.
2. With the power of speech it is quite different. This develops more and more during evolution and it only comes into being when two things have been

internalised within the realm of a living body: blood and air.

3. All the lower animals live in the element of water. They hear.

   All the higher animals ascend from the water into the air. But they take the water with them in the form of blood. And when air and blood meet, they develop the power of sound.

II

1. Hearing: keeping the air away.
   Speaking: making use of the air.
2. Birds and Fishes.
   The birds sing, but are deaf.
   The fishes are silent, but hear.
   The birds separate air from blood.
   The fishes separate blood from air.
3. Human being in the equilibrium between air and blood develops the power of speech.
   Adam names creation!

III

1. The larynx.
   The anatomy of the larynx.
   Muscles, cartilage, air.
2. The fivefoldness of the larynx.
3. The physiology of the larynx.

IV

1. The two parents of speech:
   a. The Mother: hearing;
   b. The Father: muscle-movement.

thinking ⟶ hearing ⟶ larynx-structure

willing ⟶ movement ⟶ air within the larynx

2. Hearing and movement meet in the realm of blood and air and there language can incarnate.

V

1. Language is the child.
2. The larynx is the cradle.
3. The human being is Christophorus.
4. The fifth part of the larynx, the tongue!

A Study on Hearing

A study from 1953

If we want to form the right picture of hearing we must attempt to bring together a variety of world factors; only then can a first glimpse of this mystery come about.

I

Firstly, tone is self-contained, and the vibration of air is nothing but a garment that must be taken off before it reaches the inner ear ('Take off your shoes, because you are treading on holy ground.'). In this sense the outer ear, consisting of the eardrum, the auditory ossicles and the oval window, have been prepared in advance for the oncoming breath of air. Apart from this, a transformation takes place in the medium that transfers the rhythm in that the fluid area of the inner ear is formed out of the airy region in the outer and middle ear. Only the smallest hint of what was vibration on the outside reaches there.

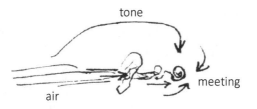

Anatomically, the structure of the inner ear corresponds to the ovaries. The Graafian follicle[1] is formed like a primitive organ of balance from which hearing initially comes about like an act of fertilisation. The remaining vibrations behave like the germ cells: they bring chaos to the inner ear like the seed disturbs the egg-cells. Chaos is brought about and within this the tone is born; it sinks down into the organ of Corti, just like the spirit germ unites with the earthly germ.

II

Next, the labyrinth of the inner ear consists of two parts: the organ of balance and the organ of hearing. The organ of balance is now known to be a metamorphosis of the tripartite blood circulation and the heart. If this is the case, the structure of the organ of hearing (saccule and cochlea, endolymphatic sac) is like a lung system that lies next to the heart and vascular organ; here the saccule corresponds to the lung, and the cochlea to a metamorphosis of the bronchial system. (In certain bird species the syrinx appears in the shape of a snail, a cochlea.) So it would then be the case that an enhanced bronchial-throat system resides in the cochlea: what first appears in evolution as the lagena corresponds to the trachea, and the organ of Corti to the larynx. Yet, it is a 'dumb' larynx, not a larynx geared for speaking but for hearing. A larynx that does not have a movement function but a receptive one.

The endolymphatic sac, however, with its indirect communication with the cerebrospinal fluid, takes up the rhythm of the breathing activity and leads it into the cochlea.

One can now see from this, that two rhythms meet in the ear in an extremely quiet way. The first one coming from the outer ear and the second expanding from the cerebrospinal fluid. But because the breathing is a cosmic sun-rhythm, this rhythm is constantly keeping both the sacculus and the utricle tuned to the cosmic sun harmony, preparing the labyrinth for hearing.

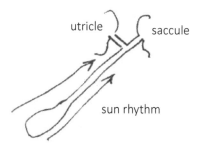

utricle   saccule

sun rhythm

endolymphatic sac

III

In relation to this, however, the following should be kept in mind. The actual apparatus that perceives sound is the muscular system in its entirety, which is directly embedded within the sound-body as a receptive organ. It is not that we 'perceive' with this receptive organ, but we do 'take in' what resounds as sound, for sound belongs to that space which may be called true space. It is the space of sunlight from which we have removed ourselves due to the formation of our sense of equilibrium, at least to the degree that we no longer go along with the movements of the earth, the sun-earth, and the earth-sun-stars taking place within it. Yet it is this space that resounds, and the limbs are embedded in it.

This music that is taken up by the limbs, and which at the same time is movement, streams through the limbs to the centre, to the heart, and from there to the lung where it is dammed up and reaches the larynx.

Through the fact that this movement impulse carrying the sounds and rhythms travels upwards and comes to a halt in the larynx, it brings about the transformation from air into sound. This is how the sound is born in its substantiality.

Giving birth to the sound out of the air is an act most intimately connected with the understanding of what is being heard.

The sound now strives upwards, changes within the space of the mouth into word and speech and thus has made a connection with the ear.

The movement that strives upwards from below is repelled, just like the stream of air vibrations striving from outside to inside is repelled.

The lower stream gives birth to the tone as its child. The upper stream is a fertilising stream.

IV

Yet now we need to keep in mind something else, namely the nerve supply to the cochlea and to the organ of balance. This nerve-supply is extraordinarily extensive and leads from the cochlear nucleus to the nucleus of the eighth nerve and from there via the tectum[2] into the temporal lobe. The connections are extremely extensive, so that they are being led into all parts of the nerve substance.

It is not hearing itself that is transmitted in this way, however, but the connection of what is heard with other sense impressions: mainly what is seen along with the sense of one's own movement. What has been heard has great difficulty to exist as something real in itself. Only if it connects with other sense impressions does it find 'itself', recognises itself as such. If this has been understood, the path will lead down from the nerves into the kidney.

About the Kidney and the Ear

Notes for a lecture in Newton Dee, April 28, 1962

Pronephros   glomerulus and main part
Mesonephros   transitionary and middle part (renal tubulus)
Metanephros   renal pelvis and urethra

In the eleventh lecture of the first doctors' course it is described how 'the Earth's coal or carbon content regulates the oxygen content of the Earth's environment'.[1] This does, however, imply a direct relationship with the process by which the animal is formed:

> The interaction between the Earth's coal-forming process and the oxygen process in the Earth's atmosphere is underlaid by a force that, to the spiritual-scientific way of looking at things, is revealed as the tendency to become animal.[2]

This could be understood to mean that only then the atmospheric foundation of animal life, the breathing, is created. Afterwards, 'etheric beings' are mentioned that 'constantly strive to escape from the Earth'.[3]

The process of light formation in the human being.
Original light.

Carbon is initially completely destroyed in the lower part of the human being, and then built up again anew.

This reanimation of carbon is connected with what manifests as the generation of light in normal human beings. This internal generation of light meets the operation of the light from the external world. Our upper organic sphere is designed so as to enable external light and internal light to counteract one another.

The breaking down of the carbon substance, however, is connected with the kidney-bladder-process.

Disgust as a symptom of animal formation leads to vomiting, and continues into coma: Uraemia!

Eclampsia.[4]

Pregnancy is an image of the process of becoming animal.

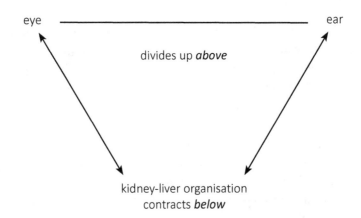

This is functionally different from what is otherwise dominant up above in the brain as a synthesising (constructive) tendency and below in the abdomen as an analysing (destructive) tendency.

About the kidney system, in the lecture of October 27, 1922.[5]

After Volhard.[6]

Nephrosclerosis The 'I', circulation
Nephritis   Astral body, breathing
Nephrosis   Etheric body, fluid system

For example, in hearing:

Nephrosclerosis Loss of tone
Nephritis   Loss of speech sound
Nephrosis   Loss of sound

In order to understand the collaboration of ear and kidney, the idea of breaking-down forces needs to be introduced. It is probably the case that the breaking-down processes taking place within the kidney make it possible that above in the ear there is the ability to hear. A sense organ must, to a certain extent, be kept free from constructive processes, and therefore a corresponding organ is needed which makes this possible. In the sense organ itself the destructive processes should not be dominant either.

It seems to be the case that the collaboration of hearing and the function of the kidney plays out in such a way that down below a strong breaking-down process occurs, while above, a hollow space – a listening space – comes about in which hearing can take place.

Apart from this something else seems to occur: while above in the ear there is hearing, down below in the kidneys, music is made.

How can this be understood?

The malpighian corpuscles are shaped like a small placenta and the Bowman's capsule resembles the amnion. A 'nourishing stream' is being extracted from the blood circulation, which then flows through the various parts of the renal tubule. There it is being scanned, and various substances are filtered back. This process of filtering back resembles a form of chemical music making.

In this way, urine is our own amniotic fluid and the kidney a placenta-like organ. We extract from our own blood so many building-up forces that, up above, we are creating the space in which we can hear but also think. Consciousness comes about through this.

In the same way that a soul-being is able to penetrate the embryonic sheaths, so are tone and thoughts able to fill the consciousness space.

The organ of day consciousness is not in the brain, but in the kidney.

These are three conditions that are closely interlinked:

Consciousness   Ear

Metanephros

Movement of the Limbs
and Cancer Prophylaxis

Notes for a lecture given in Comburg on April 13, 1953

I

1. The change in the situation since the middle of the
   [twentieth] century in relation to the study and
   understanding of Anthroposophy.
   a. On working in accordance with Rudolf Steiner's
   work.
   b. The beginning of carrying each other's destinies.
2. A contribution out of the curative educational
   experience must be given to the understanding of the
   problem of cancer.
3. A mutual carrying of the different disciplines will lead
   to grasping the truth. The joy of experiencing the truth.

II

1. The examination of deaf children produced a clear
   sign of cancer in the crystal image test. A further
   examination of the results of this test led to the
   discovery of hyperactivity of the limbs.
2. The polarity of hearing—movement of the limbs.
   Presentation with the help of R.St. Tenth lecture of *The
   Foundations of Human Existence.*[1]
3. Hypersensitivity in the hearing of cancer patients, who,
   although their sight is not so strong (Dr M. Hauschka)

are more alert in the area of the hearing than other people. The essential being of the listening space, the portal to the higher senses.

III

1. What is hearing?
   The process of cancer formation and hearing (quote by R. St.).
   The realm of the life ether.
2. What is the content of life ether?
   The sense of smell ... Life ether and consciousness soul.
   Recognition of the other person's 'I', of the 'name'.
3. Hearing is 'recognising the eternal name of things and beings.'
   Description of the process of speaking.

IV

1. The lung as an organ which is present within us as the counter image of the life ether. (Quote by R.St).
   It opens up the sense of hearing.
2. Speech process and movement.
   Lung and kidney in their mutual exchange.
3. This is how the gesture-movement was transformed within into the speech process, and thus we have forgotten how to understand the language of nature.

V

1. What is movement?
   Description of the three types of paralysis.
   Spastic – athetotic – rigid.
2. Description of the three musical forms of movement:
   Spastic – melody
   Rigid – harmony
   Athetotic – rhythm
3. Thinking movement

Speech movement
Gesture movement

VI

1. Modern civilisation as a factor in the hindrance of
   movement:
   Spastic paralysis – desk and car people
   Rigid paralysis – people are overwhelmed by noise
   Athetotic paralysis – conveyor belt people
   All this points to the disposition for cancer
2. Prophylaxis:
   Renewal of the gesture movement – eurythmy
   Renewal of the speech movement – speech formation
   Renewal of the thinking movement – inner
   development
3. In this way one could begin a cancer prophylaxis.
   Physician and patient
   The cancer patient anticipates what is not yet so visible
   in us: the separation of the life-ether from the process
   of earthly formation – Goethe.

Music and Musical Experience

I

Notes for a lecture given in Camphill, June 4, 1958

> For one who listens in stillness
> A soft, sustaining tone
> Resounds through all the tones
> In the colourful earthly dream
> *Friedrich Schlegel*

What the human being is in the realm of nature is music in the realm of sounds. Sounds are natural. Tone, however, is something new. It does not exist in the created world at all but must first be created within it. Tone can only be compared with the ego as it is taking hold of itself. The experience of tone, however, is a totally different thing. Just as I have a sense of ego, so do I also experience tone with the whole of the human being, but without the sense organisation.

Nerve-organisation
Rhythmic system $\Big\}$ they experience the tone
Movement organism

I

There are various reasons why we are now beginning to speak about the musical aspects.

The preliminaries:

1. The need to write something about music and curative education. This made me aware of how incomplete and insufficient music therapy is that is being practised in the world at present. Yet, at the same time, I was also able to experience how completely insufficient our own attempts are that we have so far undertaken.

2. The way we have occupied ourselves with the origin of the musical instruments in order to come again a little closer to musical life.

   Then there was also a study of a number of comments by Rudolf Steiner about music in present and future times, resulting in a number of findings and the determination to once more and perhaps in a much more intensive way than before come closer to the element of music.

II

1. Contemporary music therapy:
   America and Sweden. Examples of Pontvik and Podolsky.

2. Our own music therapy:
   Simplification
   The tone itself should do it.

Treatment for the hearing impaired and for paralysis: should have been tone.

   Music therapy for pre-psychosis and post encephalitis: rhythm.

III

1. Musical instruments:
   Development of humankind
   Dionysian-Apollonian

2. Musical experience today:

Quote from the Torquay course
Goetheanum
Modern painting
Modern sculpture

IV

1. R. Steiner: Remarks from September 29, 1920 (Reply to a question).
   Tone as something that exists within itself, that wants to be freed up in order to be able to resound by itself.
   Tone-sound / ego-nature

noises	physical
sounds	etheric
speech sound	astral
tones	ego

   Tone is not something that is present in the world. It is only being brought into the world.

2. R. Steiner: Lecture of March 7, 1923, last sentence:
   'Only a truly irrational understanding – an understanding of the human being beyond the rational...'[1]

Sentence on the first page:
   There is a tone-physiology for sounds!
   There is no tone-physiology for tones![2]

For this reason we have been occupying ourselves with this for many years now and still we have not really been understood.

II

Notes for a lecture given in Camphill, June 11, 1958

I

1. After having discussed the preliminaries towards an understanding of the musical element, today we would like to venture a bit further into the realm of the audible. Therefore we will again put before us Rudolf Steiner's sentence from his lecture of March 7, 1923: 'that tone physiology does not really have anything to say about the musical element ... There is only a tone physiology for sounds; there is no tone physiology for tones.'[3]

2. It becomes clear from this sentence that R. Steiner gives a totally different value, a different significance to tone than to sound. He also only speaks about speech sound in connection to language and makes a distinction between tone-eurythmy and speech-eurythmy. And here we return to our four stages of hearing:

> Noise
> Sound
> Speech sound
> Tone

We would like to occupy ourselves again with this subdivision. We called it the 'members of hearing'. They are assigned to what is heard, to the ear as a sense-organ, yet we are dealing here with something different from mere members of one area of the senses.

3. In tasting, for instance, I distinguish four or seven qualities: sweet, sour etc. But this is a totally different sequence from the one we meet here. Here we see

stages of development, and we would like to find out how to grasp this:

Noise

Noise is that which is present as continuous background to all we hear. Just as the sense of touch is the foundation for all sense experiences in that it forms the ground of our existence, so is noise the presence which pervades our listening space and never ever leaves it.

Noise can be amplified and become din, it can become thundering and roaring. It can become so overpowering that it can make our body shake even as far as inducing death.

If we wish to explain it, we must say that noise can be attributed to anything that is material, in as far as it moves within earthly space.

Something quite different, however, comes towards us when we speak about sound.

Sound

Sound is a much more inward and more harmonious process. In sound, noise has been clarified in the way a mineral or a different kind of substance turns into a crystal. Graphite is noise. Sound is of the same substance as diamond. Each sound has, as its main state of existence, form and this is why it appears to be transparent.

A similar process can be found in a different area: for example, if the manifold types of smells and scents turn into the spectrum of taste, or if greyness is transformed into a colour spectrum.

noise	variations of greyness
sound	colours
speech sound	images
tone	

Sound permeates all creation, both inorganic and organic. The world of sounds helps to build all matter. Chemistry. One does not always have to hear the world of sounds, but it may be heard.

sense of touch	noise
sense of life	sound

Every instrument resounds. It also has tones and yet these tones are in the first instance only sounds. Any mathematical law of tones, as high or low, in connection with the frequencies, the length of the strings etc, belongs to the area of sound.

Speech sound

This is again something new. Noise is an illogical mixture of sounds. Speech sound, however, is a logical arrangement of various sounds.

Here the overtones come to the fore more strongly and surround and enhance the sound. A speech sound only comes about where the life of soul reveals itself. A tree can resound inwardly but the spirit of the tree is only able to manifest itself in speech sounds.

Language is built up out of speech sounds. The speech sound has only one organic correspondence: the muscle. This is built up out of sounds, out of tissue.

sense of touch	noise
sense of life	sound
sense of movement	speech sound

Tone

Only tone arises from the spirit depths; it is again something completely new, and only appears under quite particular conditions.

'Though I speak with the tongues of men or of angels and I have not love, then my speaking remains like sounding brass or tinkling cymbal' (1Cor 13).

II

1. The condition for the appearance of tone, however, is the world of music. Yet what does this mean?

sense of touch	noise
sense of life	sound
sense of movement	speech sound
sense of balance	tone

In the sense of balance, we no longer experience only our own body: here, the self begins to orientate with the body in the world. So, two cooperating entities are necessary: the world and the self within the body.

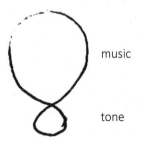

music

tone

For tone, the world of music is needed. It is manifested through tone and tone through it.

It is only through tone that the world of music is born; only through tone does it become manifest.

From [Rudolf Steiner's] lecture of December 2, 1922, 'Human utterance through tone and word':

On earth, we can speak and sing only by means of air, and in the air formations of the tone element we have an earthly reflection of a soul-spiritual element. This soul-spiritual element of tone belongs in reality to the super-sensible world, and what lives here in the air is basically the body of tone. It is not surprising, therefore, that one rediscovers tone in the spiritual world.[4]

2. What is the 'world of music'? What appears when a note really resounds? Becoming a true note can only be done together with other notes. Yet that which lives in between the notes, between that which is heard today, this alone is music. The intervals between the notes, this is music. The true melos, this is music.
   Quotation from *Eurythmy as Visible Singing*: 'Where does the musical element really lie...'[5]

3. Yet with this we have achieved a very first grasp of the field of music. It is that which spans between the notes. Here we should not imagine notes like poles that have been rammed into the 'air' earth with the garlands and chains of the intervals winding in between them.
   The notes are like human 'egos', appearing as personalities ('personare' is Latin for sounding through). In the relationship that comes about between them, in their meeting and parting, in their coming and going, in all that we may call contact, we have an image of that which also works through the power of music. Every tone is an 'ego'- point which forms a connection with other 'egos'.
   The mutual relationship of the notes to each other, their sociology, is the musical element. Yet this arises, becomes and is found on earth through the fact that we human beings can set the tone outside ourselves.

III

1. Now, however, we are coming to the question: 'How does the musical element, which is already sense-free in that it is not heard, become experience? How can we, nevertheless, sense it?' And the question goes further: 'How and where do we experience noise, sound and speech sound if there is no tone or the music belonging to it?'
Rudolf Steiner's indication in the lecture of March 7, 1923:

> The ear is important to the musician only in so far as it is in the position of experiencing, without having a relationship to the outer world such as the eye has, for instance ... the musical experience is really an experience of the whole human being.[6]

2. The ear as sense organ only begins its development with the vertebrates.
Fishes: lateral lines
Rhythmical sensations of touch
The entire nervous system connected with the utricle, except the motoric nerves, senses noise.
The ear is the organ for sounds.
The ear and the larynx hear speech sounds.
The senses of word and of thought, however, stream into this as a transformation of the senses of movement and of life.
Music and tone are sensed by the so-called motoric nervous system, are lifted upwards by the breath and reflected by the ear as a sound structure. Resonance is not the actual experience, but only the stimulus for the experience.
3. Within these conclusions, however, there is already much that can lead to therapy.

Noise: for the enlivening of touch
Sounds: for the ear itself.
Speech sounds: for the larynx, speech problems etc.
Melos: for the whole of the human being, but
                especially for those who move too
                strongly, or for those who are unable
                to move.

4. Harmony and rhythm are the first to attach themselves
to melos. This, however, can be called 'gradually
becoming unmusical'. Nevertheless, contemporary
music and the experience of music are not possible
without beat and rhythm.

Next time we will speak about the intervals being the
essence of music.

III

Notes for a lecture given in Camphill, June 18, 1958

Last time we said that it is true that the entire nervous
system senses noise, but that the manifestation of this
sensory part of the nervous system is the skin and, in
connection with this, the outer ear, the eardrum, the little
auditory bones (ossicles) and in fact all that has a vibrating
nature.

On the one hand, the eye comes about from the skin in
as far as it becomes cornea. A brightening occurs.

On the other hand, the ear also comes from the skin in
as far as it becomes eardrum. Elasticity and tension occur.
In the eye the lens connects to the cornea.

In the ear the apparatus of the auditory ossicles connects

to the eardrum. And yet, just as the eye itself is not seen when light penetrates it, in the same way the ear is not heard when noise is experienced.

The next thing is the experience of sound. This takes place in the cochlea, in the actual ear. This experience as sensation, however, must be able to lift itself away from a background. It must, so to speak, be possible to be experienced because it can stand out against something else and sound more strongly than something else. The background is here the cerebrospinal fluid because it carries within itself the rhythms of pulse and breathing. This is the screen, the grid by which all sound can be perceived.

Therefore, we have here the organ of Corti, together with the streaming of the lymph in the inner ear, which hits upon the resonance box of the meningeal sac via the endolymphatic sac.

In the eye colour is equivalent to sound. With the help of the retina a sensation of colour is revealed from undifferentiated light, just as the organ of Corti only transmits sounds.

The next step is the experience of speech sounds and thus also the experience of hearing language. This takes place in such a way that the background of the cerebrospinal fluid fades out, because the keynote is getting lost and all the overtones arise. This causes a strong noise element to enter the sound, but the larynx as organ is now connected with the ear [sic] and this anchor gives the possibility to perceive the speech sound. Something form-like now occurs.

In relation to the eye, this step is taken in that the optic nerve extends to the brain and reaches further unto the occipital lobe and then is extended further. This forms a similar anchor for the formation of form and shape, as the larynx does for the speech sound.

The metamorphosis from larynx to the occipital bone also points to this.

Finally, we come to tone. Here, however, it is the entire complex of motor nerves that must be considered the sensory organ. Here is expressed the all-embracing element of the world of tone, which is a totally supersensible being, higher than the human being.

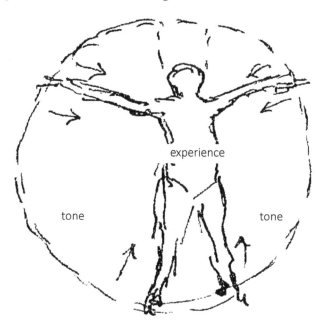

The all-embracing element of the world of tone

In the eye this can only be compared with the fact that I can look another person 'in the eye' and thus find their soul. Yet this is as far as any form of sense experience of seeing goes.

In hearing, however, music only begins with the experience of tone, because the interval arises, manifests, comes into being between the tones. And the real musical experience is the actual interval, the interplay between the 'I' and the other bodies. The 'I' corresponds to the tone:

the relationships and cooperation between 'I' and the rest of the members of the organism, especially the soul and the spirit, are the intervals.

seventh	I	atman
sixth	I	buddhi
fifth	I	manas
		consciousness soul,
fourth	I	intellectual soul,
		sentient soul
third	I	astral body – minor,
		ether body – major
prime	I	physical body

Here lies the reason why Rudolf Steiner always referred to the history of humanity when he had been speaking about the intervals.

Atlantis		seventh	
Transition	Indian		
	Persian	sixth	
Egyptian-Chaldean		fifth	
Graeco-Latin		fourth	
Since 1500 or 1600		third	major
			minor

Someone who craves oxygen:	experience of minor
Someone who longs to release carbon dioxide:	experience of major

The ether body pushes back the astral body.

This is where all contemporary musical experience originates, for the way we experience the intervals is different from before. In his lecture of March 8, 1923, Rudolf Steiner said about the experience of the fifth and the fourth:

> [Human beings] required no instrument in order to
> produce outwardly the interval of a fifth ... Then the
> experience of the fourth was also lost. One required an
> outer instrument so one could be objectively certain of
> the fourth.[7]

And at the end of this lecture he says:

> When he built physical musical instruments, man simply
> filled the empty spaces that remained after he no longer
> beheld the spiritual. Into those spaces he put the physical
> instruments.[8]

All our contemporary music is totally [connected] to
the experience of the third coming about from the lower
self of the human being when inhaling and exhaling.
The imaginations of the intervals are generated by the
instruments and remind us of how things used to be.

Music is 'Spirit Recollection'.

From the major and minor third as an experience, that
is the harmony permeated by minor and major, music rises
upwards with the breathing and becomes melody and it
moves downwards with the beat of heart and pulse and
becomes rhythm. Thus, all that is musical again resonates
with the human form and finds itself there.

The instruments replace the experience of the spirit;
the intervals remind one of the paths of initiation, and
sometimes at special moments a first inkling resounds in
a piece by Bruckner or Mahler of what will one day again
come to be.

Movement and Hearing

Notes for a lecture given in Brachenreuthe, May 1, 1960

I

1. A year ago we spoke about agriculture and its inner
   content. This time the theme that was proposed is
   'Movement and Hearing'. This is warranted for a home
   for children with movement disorders.
2. For many years one of my most profound concerns has
   been to research the issue of hearing and movement,
   to understand the extraordinary construction of the ear
   and to grasp the world of movement.

   Looking into it more closely we find that we are not
   dealing with isolated phenomena in either, but with
   processes connected with the *totality* of our structure, of
   the body, the soul and the spirit.

   We *hear* with the whole of our organism. We move with
   the whole of our organism.
3. Hearing as an overall experience.

   We react to sounds and tones as a whole organism.
   With the totality of our rhythmical system – heart-
   circulation-breathing – we are a soundbox for the
   experiences of sound that flow around us. The organ of
   vibrations of Katz and Révesz.
4. Movement as an overall human phenomenon.

   Buytendijk's book. The expression of the soul in
   movement. Gestures, mimicry, emotions.
   The language of movement of blind children.

The expressive movements of deaf children.
The incomplete movements of children with impaired movement.

II

1. The structure of the organism
   The head as resting.
   The chest as rhythmical.
   The limbs as moving.
   Description of the confinement within the head (fingers and toes = teeth).
   The opening up in the chest.
   The liberation in the limbs.
2. The ear lives in the resting head.
   About the shape of the ear.
   Eardrum, the auditory ossicles.
   Paralysed, hardened organ.
   The tone *sinks into* the movement, and is *resurrected* in the ear.
3. If one goes a stage deeper, we come across language; musical sound, speech sound and movement are blended together here. Speech is not possible without the movement of the larynx-organisation.
   Anatomy of the larynx: a torso without limbs, but limbs are continually being created as a resounding structure in the act of speaking. The rhythmical organisation as seedbed and bed for speech.
4. In the limbs the sound dies and becomes movement.
   Movement itself becomes a musical phenomenon; it cannot be heard but can be experienced and seen.
   What is involuntary movement?
   What is concealed within all movement?
   The false concept of the motor nerves.

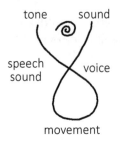

III

1. About the analysis of movement:
    a. The intention: taking hold, embracing, repelling, pushing, rushing, GOAL.
    b. The tension between myself and the goal is the melody.
    c. My 'being in tune' determines the harmony of the movement.
    d. Predisposition and temperament; the course of the movement, the beat, i.e. the rhythm.
2. Melody, harmony and beat are the basic principles of all musical laws.
   It is always the whole human being.
   Moving = speaking.
   Dancing = singing.

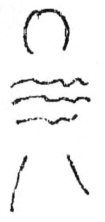

melody

harmony

beat

3. A continuous sounding and moving streams through us. It comes out of a tone-world that surrounds us and is simultaneously in movement and constantly emerging.

Die Sonne tönt nach alter Weise
In Brudersphären Wettgesang.
Und ihre vorgeschrieb'ne Reise
Vollendet sie mit Donnergang.

The sun-orb sings, in emulation,
Mid brother-spheres, his ancient round:
His path predestined through creation
He ends with step of thunder-sound.[1]

4. The words of St Basil: 'The body is a string instrument (psaltery), intended for the singing of hymns, to our God. The actions of the body can themselves become psalms, because the body has itself been created so harmoniously that even our movements become harmony.'[2]
The words of Saint-Martin: 'The human being is like a lyre of God.'[3]

Notes

Introduction
Translated by Edeline LeFevre

1. Bertha König, 'Meine Kindheits- und Lebenserinnerungen' [Recollections of My Life], Karl König Archive, Aberdeen. Unpublished document, translated by Robin Jackson, 2010.
2. Diary entry by Karl König, July 1918.
3. See Anne Weise, 'Anekdoten aus dem musikalischen Leben Karl Königs' [Anecdotes from Karl König's Musical Life], *Newsletter of the Karl König Institute*, No.13, Summer 2015.
4. The moon node refers to the moment when the moon returns to the constellation it was in at the time of an individual's birth. This occurs once every 18 years and 7 months. It can be a time of deepened self-knowledge and decisive achievements. More deeply hidden life impulses and tasks are recognised and a transition to a new phase in life takes place.
5. König, *At the Threshold to the Modern Age*, pp. 369–83.
6. From a telephone conversation between the author and Christof-Andreas Lindenberg on July 11, 2016. König later told this story to Lindenberg when they were together in the house in Camphill where Mahler's portrait was hanging.
7. König, *Die Wissenschaft vom Lebendigen* [The Science of Living Things], a lecture given to the Institute for Embryology, Vienna, on December 3, 1925. From the Karl König Archive.
8. König, *My Task*, p. 19.
9. König, *Die Wissenschaft vom Lebendigen* [The Science of Living Things].
10. Although he never personally met Rudolf Steiner, König later found out that he and Steiner had been at the same concert performance of Bruckner's *Eighth Symphony* in Vienna. See Anne Weise, 'Fragments from Karl König's Life-Journey: Socialistic Youth Ideals, Anthroposophy, Building the Camphill Movement', *Newsletter of the Karl König Institute*, No. 13, Summer 2015.
11. König, *My Task*, p. 19.

12. Steiner, *Goethe's World View*, p. 49.
13. Anke Weihs, 'Life with Dr König', in *Karl König: My Task*, p. 148.
14. Hans Heinrich Engel, 'Some Personal Memories', in *Karl König: My Task*, p. 152.
15. König's Notebook, *c.* 1926.
16. König, *The Human Soul*, p. 23.
17. Ibid. p. 97.
18. Diary entry of November 28, 1954. See König, *The Seasons and Their Festivals*, p. 85.
19. These notes can be accessed on the website of the Karl König Institute (www.karlkoeniginstitute.org/en/karl-koenig-books.asp)
20. This lecture can be accessed on the website of the Karl König Institute (www.karlkoeniginstitute.org/en/karl-koenig-books.asp)
21. Eugen Kolisko (1893–1939). Physician. He discovered anthroposophy in 1914 and attended lectures by Steiner. He became the school doctor at the first Waldorf School in Stuttgart, Germany, where he worked with the teachers on preventative medicine, which also included therapeutic singing. In 1936 he emigrated to Britain with his wife, Lili, and would later play a major part in helping König gain asylum in Scotland.
22. König, *My Task*, pp. 20f.
23. Ibid. p. 28.
24. Steiner, *The Inner Nature of Music and the Experience of Tone*, p. 56. See lecture of March 7, 1923.
25. See Steel, *Art in Community – Community as Art*.
26. See Müller-Wiedemann, *Karl König*.
27. Compare Schauder, *Vienna, My Home*.
28. See website: www.uni-muenster.de/imperia/md/content/ musikpaedagogik/musiktherapie/pdf-dateien/liste_der_dissertationen_ und_habilitiationen_2017.pdf
29. Schauder, *Vienna, My Home*.
30. Ibid.
31. Compare *The Superintendent's Report of the Camphill Rudolf Steiner Schools for Children in Need of Special Care*, January 31, 1946 – January 31, 1947.
32. Andrea Rauter on May 4, 2013, in an email to John Baum, who was researching the early history of Camphill.
33. Kolisko, *Sozial therapeutischer-medizinischer Gesangskurs* [Social Therapeutic-medical Singing Course].
34. Ibid.
35. Christof-Andreas Lindenberg on Susanne Müller-Wiedemann in Surkamp, *The Lives of Camphill*.

36. Susanne Müller-Wiedemann, 'Die Hörraum-Therapie und die
Tonstärken-Therapie' [The Listening-room Therapy and the Sound-
strength Therapy], in Beilharz, *Erziehen und Heilen durch Musik*
[Educating and Healing Through Music]. Article translated and
privately published by Edeline LeFevre.

37. Susanne Müller-Wiedemann, 'Über die Anwendung von Musik
und Eurythmie in der Behandlung hör- und sprachgestörter Kinder'
[About the Use of Music and Eurythmy in the Treatment of Hearing-
and Speech-impaired Children], in Pietzner, *Aspekte der Heilpädagogik*
[Aspects of Curative Education]. (Article not included in the English
version of the book). See also, Susanne Müller-Wiedemann, 'Aus der
Arbeit mit tauben Kinder' [From working with deaf children], in *Das
Seelenpflegebedürftige Kind* [The Child with Special Needs], Easter 1955.

38. Teirich, Hildebrand Richard, *Musik in der Medizin* [Music in
Medicine]. König's article 'Music Therapy in Curative Education' was
published for the Camphill Movement in English in Pietzner, *Aspects
of Curative Education*.

39. About the therapy with coloured shadows see also Karl König, 'The
Brain-injured Child', lecture given in London on May 7, 1950.
Available at the Karl König Archive.

40. Compare Zajonc, *Catching the Light*.

41. Veronika Bay, 'Music Therapy for Handicapped Children', *British
Society for Music Therapy*, Vol. 5, No. 2, Summer 1974.

42. From Veronika Bay's obituary by Theodora Geraets.

43. About 'inner movements' see Steiner, *Man in the Light of Occultism,
Theosophy and Philosophy*, lecture of June, 11 1912, and Pfrogner, *Die
drei Lebensaspekte der Musik* [The Three Life Aspects of Music].

44. Engel, *Musical Anthropology*.

45. Steiner, *Introducing Anthroposophical Medicine*, lecture of April 3, 1920,
p. 209.

46. Ibid. p. 207.

47. Excerpts from this article are contained in this book. The entire
article can be found on the website of the Karl König Institute (www.
karlkoeniginstitute.org/en/karl-koenig-books.asp).

48. Pracht, *Einführung in das Leierspiel* [Introduction to Playing the Lyre].

49. Teirich, *Musik in der Medizin* [Music in Medicine].

50. Gisbert Husemann, 'Hildebrand Richard Teirich: Musik in der Medizin.'
In: *Beiträge zu einer Erweiterung der Heilkunst nach geisteswissenschaftlichen
Erkentnissen* [Contributions to an Expansion of the Art of Healing
Based on Findings From the Humanities]. Volume 3. Year 12, 1959.

51. Austrian Society for the Promotion of Healing through Music: The official written history of Austrian music begins with the founding of the Gesellschaft der Förderung der Musikheilkunde on November 26, 1958. Prominent representatives from the Viennese medical and music colleges were members of this Society, among others Andreas Rett (neuro-pediatrician), Hans Hof (board member of the university clinic for neurology and psychiatry), Hans Sittner and Editha Koffer-Ullrich. www.musiklexikon.ac.at/ml/musik_M/Musiktherapie.xml

52. BSMT, British Society for Music Therapy (1958–2011). This Society, a limited company, was founded by Juliette Alvin and her colleagues under the name Society for Music Therapy and Remedial Music with the aim to promote the impulse and the development of music therapy. BSMT: www.bamt.org/about-british-association-for-music-therapy/history.html

53. Alfred Schmölz (1921–95). Music therapist and piano teacher at what was then the Academy, later the College, and presently the University for Music and the Arts in Vienna.

54. Manuela Schwartz, 'Einzelne Pioniere oder gewachsenes Netzwerk? Versuch einer historischen Eingrenzung der Geschichte der Musiktherapie' [Individual Pioneers or a Network that has Grown? An Attempted Historic Delineation of the History of Music Therapy]. Lecture given at the conference 'Thirty Years German Society for Music Therapy', on September 17, 2004.

55. See 'Correspondence between Hildebrand Richard Teirich and Karl König' in this volume.

56. In the German language there are different words for sound meaning musical sound which in German is *Klang* and sound meaning speech sound which in German is *Laut*. In this book, 'sound' is used for *Klang* and 'speech sound' for *Laut*.

The Word, Singing and Speaking as Revelation of the Soul
Translated by Richard Steel

1. Steiner, *The Inner Nature of Music and the Experience of Tone*, lecture of December 2, 1922, pp. 32f.

2. Morgenstern, Christian, 'Im Baum, du liebes Vöglein dort' [You Dear Bird in Yonder Tree]. Translated by Richard Steel.

3. Steiner, *The Cycle of the Year*, lecture of April 4, 1923, pp. 71f.

4. Ibid., lecture of April 3, 1923, pp. 58f.

5. See the essay 'The Four Stages of Hearing' in this volume.

6. Steiner, *Man and the World of the Stars*, p. 184.

7. From the third verse of the Foundation Stone Meditation.

Musical Instruments

1. Steiner, *The Inner Nature of Music and the Experience of Tone*, lecture of March 8, 1923.
2. Steiner, *Eurythmy as Visible Singing*, lectures of February 19 and 21, 1924.
3. The aulos was a single- or double-reed pipe, usually played in pairs during the Classical period (*c.* 510–323 BC).
4. Steiner, *The Cycle of the Year*, pp. 58f. See also description in previous lecture in this volume.
5. Steiner, *Christ and the Spiritual World*, p. 68.
6. Steiner, *The Christ-Impulse*, lecture of October 25, 1909.
7. Steiner, *Christ and the Spiritual World*, lecture of December 30, 1913.

Music in Curative Education

1. König's article 'Music Therapy in Curative Education' was later published in English for the Camphill Movement in Pietzner, *Aspects of Curative Education*.
2. Steiner, *The Inner Nature of Music and the Experience of Tone*, lectures of March 7 and 8, 1923.
3. Steiner, *Eurythmy as Visible Singing*, lecture of February 21, 1924.
4. Hans Kayser (1891–1964) was a German art and music theorist and the founder of modern harmonic research.
5. Steiner, *The Inner Nature of Music and the Experience of Tone*, p. 47: 'It is widely admitted that there is a tone physiology only for sounds; there is none for tones.'

On Seeing and Hearing
Translated by Edeline LeFevre

1. Crest or ridge, as on the top of a bone.
2. The otolith are calcium carbonate crystals in the vestibular system of the inner ear.
3. The mature ovarian follicle at the final stage of development.
4. The tear ducts.

The Four Stages of Hearing
Translated by Edeline LeFevre

1. König refers to the theme he discussed in 1958 in an article 'Bewegungsgestalten und Klanggebilde. Über die Wurzel der eurythmischen Gebärden' [Movement Forms and Tonal Pictures: Concerning the Root of the Eurythmy Gestures], *Die Drei,* 1958, no 5 (not yet translated).

2. It could be that König made a mistake here. The range given for human hearing is 20Hz to 20,000Hz.

3. See Rohracher, *Mechanische Mikroschwingungen des menschlichen Körpers* [Mechanical Micro-vibrations of the Human Body].

4. Ferdinand Scheminsky (1899–1973), Austrian electrophysiologist. See *Die Welt des Schalls* [The World of Sound].

5. See Steiner, *Truth and Knowledge* and *The Philosophy of Freedom* for a more in-depth study of this theme.

6. Hauptman, *Till Eulenspiegel.*

7. Kayser, *Vom Klang der Welt* [Of the Sound of the World]. See also Kayser, *Akroasis: The Theory of World Harmonics.*

8. See Steiner, *Riddles of the Soul.*

9. See Straus, *The Primary World of the Senses.*

10. Steiner, *The Inner Nature of Music and the Experience of Tone,* p. 49.

11. See David Katz and Géza Révész, 'Musikgenuss bei Gehörlosen' [How the Deaf Enjoy Music], *Zeitschrift für Psychologie,* Vol. 99, Issue 5/6, 1926.

12. Révész, *Introduction to the Psychology of Music.*

13. Ibid.

14. Wolfgang von Buddenbrock, 'Vergleichende Physiologie' [Comparative Psychology], in *Sinnesphysiologie,* Vol. 1, Switzerland 1952.

15. Martin Hans Christian Knudsen (1871–1949), Danish physicist and oceanographer.

16. Scheminsky, *Die Welt des Schalls* [The World of Sound].

17. Steiner, *A Psychology of Body, Soul, and Spirit,* lecture of October 26, 1909, pp. 35f.

18. Lullies and Ranke, *Lehrbuch der Physiologie in zusammenhängenden Einzeldarstellungen* [Textbook of Physiology in the Context of Individual Representations]. See chapter on the physiology of hearing.

19. Steiner, *The Inner Nature of Music and the Experience of Tone,* p. 47.

20. See note 18 in this chapter.

21. Steiner, *Balance in Teaching,* lecture of September 21, 1920.

22. Kayser, *Bevor die Engel sangen* [Before the Angels Sang].

23. Louis Claude de Saint-Martin (1743–1803), French philosopher, Freemason and mystic.

24. Kassner, *Die Moral der Musik* [The Morality of Music].

Music Therapy in Curative Education

1. Quoted by Pierre Pichot in 'The Effect of Rhythm and Functional Music on Mental Defectives', *Mental Health,* Vol. 9, No. 1, August 1949.

2. Heller, *Grundriss der Heilpädagogik* [Outline of Curative Education].

3. A good overview is given in the thirty-two essays of Podolsky's anthology, *Music Therapy*.

4. See, for example, Sidney D. Mitchell and Arthur Zanker, 'Musical Styles and Mental Disorders', *Occupational Therapy and Rehabilitation*, Vol. 28, No. 5, Oct. 1949.

5. See Pontvik, *Grundgedanken zur psychischen Heilwirkung der Musik* [Basic Ideas About the Psychological Healing Effects of Music], and *Heilen durch Musik* [Healing Through Music].

6. See Pontvik, *Heilen durch Musik* [Healing Through Music].

7. Kayser, *Vom Klang der Welt* [Of the Sound of the World]. See also *Akroasis: The Theory of World Harmonics*.

8. Kayser, *Harmonia Plantarum* [Harmony of Plants].

9. Steiner, *The Inner Nature of Music and the Experience of Tone*, lecture of March 7, 1923.

10. See Edmund Pracht, 'Die Entwicklung des Musikerlebens in der Kindheit' [The Development of Musical Life in Childhood], *Erziehungskunst* [The Art of Education], Vol. 18, No. 11/12, December 1954.

11. The most important indications can be found in the lectures Steiner gave on tone eurythmy in 1924, *Eurythmy as Visible Singing*.

12. See Goethe's *Tonlehre* [Tone Theory].

13. See Steiner, *Balance in Teaching*, lecture of September 16, 1920.

14. David Katz and Géza Révész, 'Musikgenuss bei Gehörlosen' [How the Deaf Enjoy Music], *Zeitschrift für Psychologie* [Journal of Psychology], Vol. 99, Issue 5/6, 1926. See also the chapter about receptive and productive musical performance of hearing-impaired in Révész, *Introduction to the Psychology of Music*.

15. Julia Bort, 'Die Musik in der heilpädagogischen Praxis' [Music in Curative Education], *Nature*, Vol. 2, No. 1, July 1927.

16. Pracht, *Einführung in das Leierspiel* [Introduction to Playing the Lyre], Book 4.

17. For more detailed remarks on this topic see Hans Heinrich Engel, Karl König and Hans Müller-Wiedemann, 'Über schwere Kontakt-störungen im Kindesalter und deren Behandlung mit der Substanz Thalamos' [Severe Contact Disorders in Childhood and their Treatment with the Substance Thalamos], in *Der Merkurstab* [The Wand of Mercury], 60. Jhrg., Vol. 6, 2007.

18. For more information see *The Superintendent's Report*, The Camphill Rudolf Steiner Schools, 1955.

19. See Collis, *A Way of Life for the Handicapped Child*.

20. See the chapter 'Music Therapy' in Cardwell, *Cerebral Palsy: Advances in Understanding and Care*.

21. König, 'Some Aspects of the Treatment of Cerebral Palsy', *British Journal of Physiotherapy*, Vol. 7, No. 5, May 1955. See also, 'Einige Gesichtspunkte für die Behandlung gehirngelähmter Kinder' ['Some Aspects for the Treatment of Brain-paralysed Children'], *Das Seelenpflege-bedürftige Kind* [The Child with Special Needs], Year 2, Vol. 1, Michaelmas 1955.

22. Quoted in Goldstein, *Problems of the Deaf*.

23. See the summary by Edith Whetnall, 'The Deaf Child' in *The Practitioner*, Vol. 144, April 1955.

24. See *The Superintendents Report,* The Camphill Rudolf Steiner Schools, 1955. See also, Susanne Müller-Wiedemann, 'Aus der Arbeit mit Tauben' [Working with Deaf Children], in *Das Seelenpflegebedürftige Kind* [The Child with Special Needs], Year 1, Vol. 2, Easter 1955.

The Lyre

From The Cresset, The Journal of the Camphill Movement, Christmas, *Vol. II, No 2, 1955.*

1. Classical Greek performance of epic poetry.

2. Pracht, *Einführung in das Leierspiel* [Introduction to Playing the Lyre], Book 4.

Music Therapy for Deaf and Hearing-Impaired Children

1. Steiner, *The Inner Nature of Music and the Experience of Tone,* see lectures of March 7 and 8, 1923.

Deafness in Children

Translated by Edeline LeFevre.

1. Wolfgang Thiele, 'Über den Karzinomtypus' [About the Carcinoma Type], in *Deutsche medizinische Wochenschrift* [German Medical Weekly], Vol. 74, 915, 1949.

2. Steiner, *Introducing Anthroposophical Medicine*, lecture of April 3, 1920, p. 209.

3. Ibid., p. 207.

4. The images, as well as the description of the findings of the crystallisation pictures and the crystallisations themselves, were carried out by Katherine Castelliz.

5. Gisbert Husemann, 'Das Tumorproblem in Pathologie und Erziehung' [Tumors in Pathology and Education], in *Der Beitrag der*

Geisteswissenschaft zur Erweiterung der Heilkunst [The Contribution of Spiritual Science to the Art of Healing], Vol. 1, Dornach 1950.

6. Steiner, *Introducing Anthroposophical Medicine*, lecture of March 31, 1920, pp. 167f.

7. Ibid., lecture of March 31, 1920, pp. 168f.

8. Ibid., lecture of March 31, 1920, pp. 168f.

9. See Wittmaak, *Über die normale und pathologische Pneumatisation des Schläfenbeins* [The Normal and Pathological Pneumatisation of the Temporal Bone].

10. Only in birds does a separation of the lagena from the saccule take place. In reptiles the separation is indicated very precisely, and in the amphibians there only exists an enlarged saccule. Fish almost completely lack the lagena. See Ihle, et al. *Vergleichende Anatomie der Wirbeltiere* [Comparative Anatomy of Vertebrates].

11. Steiner, *Rosicrucianism and Modern Initiation*, lecture of April 22, 1924, p. 136.

12. Steiner, *Materialism and the Task of Anthroposophy*, lecture of May 5, 1921, p. 249.

13. Hass, *Karzinom und Entzündung im Rahmen allgemeinbiologischen Geschehens: Der Versuch einer Synthese* [Carcinoma and Inflammation in the Context of General Biological Events: an Attempt at Synthesis].

Music Therapy Conferences
Translated by Edeline LeFevre

1. Katarina Seeherr, Das Merkurbad [The Mercury Bath] in *Rundbrief für Musiktherapie auf anthroposophischer Grundlage* [Newsletter for an Anthroposophical Music Therapy], No. 7, March 1994.

2. Image courtesy of Edition Mensch und Musik.

3. Steiner, *Michael's Mission*, lecture of November 30, 1919, pp. 88f.

4. Talking about the columns of the first Goetheanum, Rudolf Steiner refers to the relation of the evolution from Saturn to Venus to the intervals: 'Just as the rainbow has seven colours and the musical scale seven tones from the prime to the octave – the octave is a repetition of the prime – so do we have seven columns.' See *Rosicrucianism Renewed*, p. 4. König refers also to the seven life processes in this context. Rudolf Steiner also relates the fifth to breathing in *The Inner Nature of Music and the Experience of Tone,* in the lecture of March 7, 1923. Hermann Pfrogner later takes this as a starting point to describe the connection to the life processes and talks about this to Karl König (see the correspondence between König and Pfrogner and Pfrogner, *Die*

Sieben Lebensprozesse.
5. Verse from the Rigveda in Steiner, *Egyptian Myths and Mysteries*, lecture of September 8, 1908, pp. 67f.
6. Steiner, *The Inner Nature of Music and the Experience of Tone*, lecture of December 2, 1922.
7. Steiner, *Understanding Healing*, p. 203.
8. See above, note 21 of 'Introduction'.

A Music Conference in Camphill
From The Cresset, Journal of the Camphill Movement, *Vol. VIII, No. 3, Easter 1962*
1. Anny von Lange was born in 1887 in Mühlhausen in Thüringen. As a music-scientist she prepared the ground for a lot of research within anthroposophical music therapy with her lectures and writings in her two-part work *Mensch, Musik und Kosmos* [Man, Music and Cosmos]. A fundamental idea is the development of the twelve out of the seven: the development of the chromatic scale from the seven basic tones. Related to this is her research into the connections between the planets and the tones of the diatonic scale on the one hand, and the connection between the zodiac and the tones of the chromatic scale on the other. She died in 1959 in Arlesheim near Basel.

Therapy with Music and Coloured Shadows
1. The entire article can be found on the website of the Karl König Institute (www.karlkoeniginstitute.org/en/karl-koenig-books.asp).

Correspondence Between Hildebrand Richard Teirich and Karl König
Translated by Edeline LeFevre
1. The correspondence presented here between Karl König and Hildebrand Richard Teirich is incomplete. The entire correspondence as it is held in the Karl König Archive can be found on the website of the Karl König Institute (www.karlkoeniginstitute.org/en/karl-koenig-books.asp).
2. See, for example, Pache and Bort, *Heilende Erziehung* [Healing Education].
3. Here Pracht uses the term *musikalischer Phänomenenkreis*. A more literal translation would be 'circle of musical phenomena'.
4. Peter Selg writes: 'König was excluded from the General Anthroposophical Society in 1935; this followed intensive debate and inner struggle on his part, but also after attacks on his character and

misjudgments regarding his chosen path that soon arose after his first public appearances within anthroposophical circles. König came to the anthroposophical movement as a solitary individual and an outsider, with burning social concerns and questions. His powerful presence, however, already evident in the early lectures and essays, asked too much of the established anthroposophical context and its capacities for "integration".' From *Karl König's Path into Anthroposophy*, p. 14. Karl König was readmitted to the Anthroposophical Society on June 11, 1948.

5. Subsequent letters of December 10 and 16, 1958, are about the preparation of the visit and the lecture after Easter 1959.

Correspondence Between Hermann Pfrogner and Karl König
Translated by Edeline LeFevre

1. Pfrogner, *Leben und Werk* [Life and Work], p. 6.
2. Jacobeit, *Die Enharmonik ist der ganze Mensch* [The Enharmonic is the Whole Person].
3. Pfrogner, *Leben und Werk* [Life and Work], pp. 12f.
4. Johann Nepomuk David (1895–1977). Austrian composer.
5. Fritz Büchtger (1903–78). German composer and director of the Studio for New Music and the Youth Musical School in Munich.
6. Steiner, *Man in the Light of Occultism, Theosophy and Philosophy*, pp. 170–74.
7. Christophorus was the Camphill community at Bosch en Duin, Netherlands. In what follows, the phrase 'friends in Camphill' refers to this community.
8. 'Clinic' was the name König gave to the diagnostic work done within a team of physicians and other staff.
9. See 'The Three Pillars of the Camphill Movement' in König, *The Spirit of Camphill*.
10. Pfrogner, *Leben und Werk* [Life and Work], pp. 33f.
11. Pfrogner, *Die sieben Lebensprozesse* [The Seven Life Processes].
12. Letter from König to Pfrogner, February 19, 1964.
13. This and further letters can be found in their entirety on the website of the Karl König Institute (www.karlkoeniginstitute.org/en/karl-koenig-books.asp).
14. The Camphill community in County Down, Northern Ireland.
15. Steiner, *True and False Paths in Spiritual Investigation*, lecture of August 22, 1924, pp. 220f.
16. These copies contain Pfrogner's remarks on the inner movements and

the intervals, published in his *Die drei Lebensaspekte der Musik* [The Three Life Aspects of Music].

17. Pfrogner is referring here to the Camphill school Perceval in St Prex, Vaude, Switzerland.

18. At Munich, König gave a lecture on June 14, 1965, called 'Therapeutic Village Communities for Young People and Adults in Need of Special Care'.

19. Pfrogner, *Lebendige Tonwelt* [Living World of Sound].

A Study on Hearing
Translated by Edeline LeFevre

1. The ovarian follicles, sometimes called Graafian follicles, are rounded enclosures for the developing ova in the cortex near the surface of the ovary.

2. The tectum is part of the midbrain involved in certain reflex responses relating to visual and auditory stimuli.

About the Kidney and the Ear
Translated by Edeline LeFevre

1. Steiner, *Introducing Anthroposophical Medicine*, lecture of March 31, 1920, p. 161.

2. Ibid., pp. 161f.

3. Ibid., p. 162.

4. Eclampsia means that a pregnant woman suffering from pre-eclampsia or high blood pressure has seizures during pregnancy.

5. Steiner, *Physiology and Healing*.

6. Franz Volhard (1872–1950). German enterologist and doyen of nephrology.

Movement of the Limbs and Cancer Prophylaxis
Translated by Edeline LeFevre

1. Steiner, *The Foundations of Human Experience*, lecture of September 1, 1919.

Music and Musical Experience
Translated by Edeline LeFevre

1. Steiner, *The Inner Nature of Music and the Experience of Tone*, lecture of March 7, 1923, p. 59.

2. Ibid., p. 47.

3. Ibid.

4. Ibid., lecture of December 2, 1922, p. 40.

5. Steiner, *Eurythmy as Visible Singing*, lecture of February 21, 1924, p. 63.
6. Steiner, *The Inner Nature of Music and the Experience of Tone*, pp. 49f. Lecture of March 7, 1923.
7. Ibid., lecture of March 8, 1923, p. 62.
8. Ibid., lecture of March 8, 1923, p. 74.

Movement and Hearing
Translated by Edeline LeFevre

1. *Faust Part I*, 'Prologue in Heaven', 1–4. Translated by Bayard Taylor.
2. St Basil (330–79). Bishop of Caesarea Mazaca in Cappadocia, Asia Minor.
3. Louis Claude de Saint-Martin (1743–1803). French philosopher, Freemason and mystic.

Bibliography

Beilharz, Gerhard, *Erziehen und Heilen durch Musik* [Educating and Healing Through Music], Freies Geistesleben, Germany 1998.

Cardwell, Viola E., *Cerebral Palsy: Advances in Understanding and Care*, Association for the Aid of Crippled Children, USA 1956.

Collis, Eirene, *A Way of Life for the Handicapped Child: A New Approach to Cerebral Palsy*, Faber & Faber, UK 1947.

Engel, Hans Heinrich, *Musical Anthropology: Ideas for the Study of an Anthroposophical Music Therapy*, Createspace Independent Publishing Platform, USA 2013.

Goldstein, Max A., *Problems of the Deaf*, Whitefish, USA 2012.

Hass, Ernst, *Karzinom und Entzündung im Rahmen allgemein biologischen Geschehens: Der Versuch einer Synthese* [Carcinoma and Inflammation in the Context of General Biological Events: an Attempt at Synthesis], Barth, Leipzig, Germany 1942.

Hauptman, Gerhart, *Till Eulenspiegel*, Bertelsmann, Germany 1955.

Heller, Theodor, *Grundriss der Heilpädagogik* [Outline of Curative Education], Legare Street Press, USA 2022 (first edition 1904).

Ihle, J.E.W., Kampen, P.N. van, Niestraz, H.F., Versluys, J. *Vergleichende Anatomie der Wirbeltiere* [Comparative Anatomy of Vertebrates], Springer, Germany 1971.

Jacobeit, Iris, *Die Enharmonik ist der ganze Mensch: Briefwechsel zwischen Hermann Pfrogner und Hans Heinrich Engel* [Enharmonic is the Whole Person: Correspondence Between Hermann Pfrogner and Hans Heinrich Engel], Hochschule Magdeburg-Stendal, Germany 2016.

Kassner, Rudolf, *Die Moral der Musik* [The Morality of Music], Insel, Germany 1923.

Kayser, Hans, *Akroasis: The Theory of World Harmonics*, Plowshare, USA 1970.

—, *Bevor die Engel sangen* [Before the Angels Sang], Schwabe, Switzerland 1953.

—, *Harmonia Plantarum* [Harmony of Plants], Schwabe, Switzerland 1943.

—, *Vom Klang der Welt* [The Sound of the World], Max Niehans, Switzerland 1937.

Kolisko, Eugen , *Sozial therapeutischer-medizinischer Gesangskurs* [Social Therapeutic-medical Singing Course], Pilgramshain, 1934.

König, Karl, *At the Threshold to the Modern Age*, Floris Books, UK 2011.

—, *The Human Soul*, Floris Books, UK 2006.

—, *An Inner Journey Through the Year: Soul Images and The Calendar of the Soul*, Floris Books, UK 2010.

—, *Karl König: My Task*, Floris Books, UK 2008.

—, *The Seasons and Their Festivals: Human, Earthly and Cosmic Rhythms*, Floris Books, UK 2023.

—, *The Spirit of Camphill: The Birth of a Movement*, Floris Books, UK 2018.

Lange, Anny von, *Mensch, Musik und Kosmos: Anregungen zu einer goetheanistischen Tonlehre* [Man, Music and Cosmos: Suggestions for a Goethean Theory of Sound], Vols. 1 and 2, Novalis, Germany 1956 and 1960.

Lullies, Hans, and Ranke, Otto F. *Lehrbuch der Physiologie in zusammen-hängenden Einzeldarstellungen* [Textbook of Physiology in Coherent Individual Presentations], Berlin, Heidelberg 2012.

Müller-Wiedemann, Hans, *Karl König: A Central-European Biography of the Twentieth Century*, Camphill Books, UK 1996.

Pache, Werner, and Bort, Julia (ed.), *Heilende Erziehung. Vom Wesen Seelenpflege-bedürftiger Kinder und deren pädagogische Förderung* [Healing Education: On the Nature of Children in Need of Care and Their Educational Support], Freies Geistesleben, Germany 1962 (first ed. 1956).

Pfrogner, Hermann, *Die drei Lebensaspekte der Musik* [The Three Life Aspects of Music], Novalis, Germany 1989.

—, *Die sieben Lebensprozesse. Eine musiktherapeutische Anregung* [The Seven Life Processes: a Music Therapy Suggestion], Die Kommenden, Germany 1978.

—, *Lebendige Tonwelt. Zum Phänomen Musik* [World of Sound: the Phenomenon of Music], Weilheim, Germany 2010.

—, *Leben und Werk: Versuch einer Lebensbeschreibung* [Life and Work: An Attempt at a Biography], Novalis, Germany 1985.

Pietzner, Carlo (ed), *Aspects of Curative Education*, Aberdeen University Press, UK 1966.

—, *Aspekte der Heilpädagogik.* Freies Geistesleben, Germany 1969.

Podolsky, Edward, *Music Therapy*, Whitefish, USA 2010.

Pontvik, Aleks, *Grundgedanken zur psychischen Heilwirkung der Musik* [Basic Ideas About the Psychological Healing Effects of Music], Rascher,

Switzerland 1948.

—, *Heilen durch Musik* [Healing Through Music], Rascher, Switzerland 1954.

Pracht, Edmund, *Einführung in das Leierspiel* [Introduction to Playing the Lyre], Book 4, Atelier für Leierbau, Germany 1955.

Révész, Géza, *Introduction to the Psychology of Music*, Dover, USA 2001.

Rohracher, Hubert, *Mechanische Mikroschwingungen des menschlichen Körpers* [Mechanical Micro-vibrations of the Human Being], Vienna 1949.

Schauder, Hans, *Vienna, My Home*, privately published, Edinburgh 2002.

Scheminsky, Ferdinand, *Die Welt des Schalls* [The World of Sound], Das Bergland, Germany 1935.

Schoen, Max and Schullian, Dorothy M., *Music and Medicine*, Henry Schuman, USA 1947.

Selg, Peter, *Karl König's Path into Anthroposophy*, Floris Books, UK 2008.

Steel, Richard, *Art in Community – Community as Art*, Karl König Institute, Germany 2022.

Steiner, Rudolf. Volume Nos refer to the Collected Works (CW).

—, *Art as seen in the Light of Mystery Wisdom* (CW 275), SteinerBooks, USA 2010.

—, *Balance in Teaching* (CW 302a), SteinerBooks, USA 2007.

—, *Christ and The Spiritual World and the Search for the Holy Grail* (CW 149), Rudolf Steiner Press, UK 2008.

—, *The Christ-Impulse and the Development of Ego-Consciousness* (CW 116), Rudolf Steiner Press, UK 2015.

—, *The Cycle of the Year as Breathing Process of the Earth* (CW 223), Anthroposophic Press, USA 1984.

—, *Egyptian Myths and Mysteries* (CW 106), Anthroposophic Press, USA 1971.

—, *Eurythmy as Visible Singing* (CW 278), Rudolf Steiner Press, UK 2019.

—, *The Foundations of Human Experience* (CW 293), SteinerBooks, USA 1996.

—, *Goethe's World View* (CW 6), Mercury Press, USA 1985.

—, *The Inner Nature of Music and the Experience of Tone* (CW 283), Anthroposophic Press, USA 1983.

—, *Introducing Anthroposophical Medicine* (CW 312), SteinerBooks, USA 2010.

—, *Man and the World of the Stars: The Spiritual Communion of Mankind* (CW 219), Anthroposophic Press, USA 1963.

—, *Man in the Light of Occultism, Theosophy and Philosophy* (CW 137), Rudolf Steiner Press, UK 1964.

—, *Materialism and the Task of Anthroposophy* (CW 204), Anthroposophic

Press, USA 1987.

—, *Michael's Mission* (CW 194), Rudolf Steiner Press, UK 2016.

—, *The Philosophy of Freedom* (CW 4), Rudolf Steiner Press, UK 2011.

—, *Physiology and Healing: Treatment, Therapy and Hygiene – Spiritual Science and Medicine* (CW 314), Rudolf Steiner Press, UK 2013.

—, *A Psychology of Body, Soul, and Spirit: Anthroposophy, Psychology, Pneumatosophy* (CW 115), SteinerBooks, USA 1999.

—, *The Riddle of Humanity* (CW 170), Rudolf Steiner Press, UK 1970.

—, *Riddles of the Soul* (CW 21), Mercury Press, USA 1996.

—, *Rosicrucianism and Modern Initiation: Mystery Centres of the Middle Ages – The Easter Festival and the History of the Mysteries* (CW 233a), Rudolf Steiner Press, UK 2020.

—, *Rosicrucianism Renewed: The Unity of Art, Science and Religion. The Theosophical Congress of Whitsun 1907* (CW 284), SteinerBooks, USA 2006.

—, *True and False Paths in Spiritual Investigation* (CW 243), Rudolf Steiner Press, UK 1985.

—, *Truth and Knowledge* (CW 3), SteinerBooks, USA 1981.

—, *Truth-Wrought Words with Other Verses and Prose Passages*, SteinerBooks, USA 2015.

—, *Understanding Healing: Meditative Reflections on Deepening Medicine through Spiritual Science* (CW 316), Rudolf Steiner Press, UK 2013.

Straus, Erwin, *The Primary World of the Senses: A Vindication of Experience*, Free Press of Glencoe, UK 1963.

Surkamp, Johannes (ed), *The Lives of Camphill*, Floris Books, UK 2007.

Teirich, Hildebrand, *Musik in der Medizin* [Music in Medicine], Fischer, Stuttgart 1958.

Wittmaak, Karl, *Über die normale und pathologische Pneumatisation des Schläfenbeins* [The normal and pathological pneumatisation of the temporal bone], Fischer, Germany 1918.

Zajonc, Arthur, *Catching the Light: The Entwined History of Light and Mind*, Oxford University Press, UK 1995.

Index

About the Editor

Katarina Seeherr trained in special education at Camphill in Aberdeen, Scotland, and singing therapy with Arnold Dorhout-Mees and she has a master's degree in music therapy. She helped to establish a new Camphill Community in Estonia and has taught music therapy internationally. She currently works as an anthroposophic music therapist in Berlin, Germany.

Karl König's collected works are being published in English by Floris Books and in German by Verlag Freies Geistesleben. They are issued by the Karl König Institute in co-operation with the Ita Wegman Institute for Basic Research into Anthroposophy. They encompass the entire, wide-ranging literary estate of Karl König, including his books, essays, manuscripts, lectures, diaries, notebooks, his extensive correspondence and his artistic works, across twelve subjects.

Karl König Archive subjects

Medicine and study of the human being
Curative education and social therapy
Psychology and education
Agriculture and science
Social questions
The Camphill movement
Christianity and the festivals
Anthroposophy
Spiritual development
History and biographies
Artistic and literary works
Karl König's biography

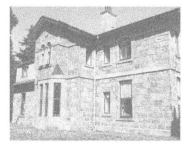

Karl König Institute
www.karlkoeniginstitute.org

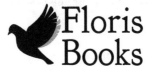

Floris Books

For news on all our **latest books,**
and to receive **exclusive discounts,**
join our mailing list at:

florisbooks.co.uk

Plus subscribers get a FREE book
with every online order!

Printed in the USA
CPSIA information can be obtained
at www.ICGtesting.com
JSHW011207050624
64305JS00002BA/2